AF737508

ineffable meaningfulness that veers towards us like a stream that runs down to us from a hidden wellspring. Where existence philosophy and existential phenomenology work at the border between the ontic and ontological language, one could say that art and certain spiritual forms of contemplative philosophy (Cooper, 2018; Hadot, 1995) work at the border between the ontological language and the pre-linguistic Being.

Pragmatic and problem-solving wonder and knowledge-seeking scientific wonder are connected to the centre of the ontic language. However, in language, deep wonder comes before thought and thought expression. Philosophical wonder would then be located in the zone of ontological language, whereas philosophical thought and expression would be found on the border between the ontic and ontological language.

Artistic wonder is far more out in the 'ocean of the ineffable' and is connected to the zone of the pre-linguistic Being and ontological and saturated silence. The artwork comes after and lives on the border between the ontological language and pre-linguistic Being.

Finally, as Patocka, Wittgenstein and Buber illuminate, we also have, as a silent horizon or source behind the pre-linguistic Being dimension, a sense of the grand mystery, which Patocka calls love or 'the force of transcendence' and Buber calls the silent Thou. Here, the meta-psychic and meta-physical phenomenon and event of love, as Buber describes it, seems germane to our ability to 'live with mystery.' In moments of deep wonder, we repeatedly experience that the world, this moment, this flower, this person, is given to us as an unexpected present and trace of something of ultimate good or, as Wittgenstein would say, with 'absolute value.' In the loving relation with the world, we sense this absolute value in the present and daily things and beings around us. A Jewish theologian and philosopher, Abraham Heschel, who has great affinity with the thinking of Martin Buber, writes:

> Finite meaning is a thought we comprehend; infinite meaning is a thought that comprehends us; finite meaning we absorb; infinite meaning we encounter. Finite meaning has clarity; infinite meaning has depth. Finite meaning we comprehend with analytical reason; to infinite meaning we respond in awe. Infinite meaning is uncomfortable, not compatible with our categories. It is not to be grasped as though it were something in the world which appeared before us. Rather it is that in which the world appears to us. It is not an object—not a self-subsistent, timeless idea or value; it is a presence. There is no insight into transcendent meaning without the premise of wonder and the premise of awe. (Heschel 1965, p. 78)

Apophatic wonder is the wonder and awe we can experience when something ineffable and, at the same time, of absolute value (a 'transcendent meaning') happens to us as a kind of epiphany or sudden gift or grace. These moments have an enduring, self-transformative and ethical impact on us in our lives.

If we compared *philosophical* wonder with *artistic* and *apophatic* (or spiritual) wonder, and used the I-Thou-philosophy of Buber (Buber, 2013/1923), one could say that the difference between 'the existential' and the 'spiritual' is that the notion of the existential is closely connected to the I in the I-Thou relation. However, the notion of the spiritual is closely connected to the Thou in the I-Thou relation. The Being dimension, about which Heidegger talks, is in the view of Buber and Patocka not identical to the existential and spiritual dimension. The Being dimension has to do with the mood and way of being (my 'being-in-the-world'), which the person is immersed into. It is *through* the Being dimension (through 'Dasein') that the human being becomes aware of the enigmatic and metaphysical I and the Otherness or alterity and transcendence of the Thou. We have, so to speak, to 'go through' the medium of Being in order to see the wonders of the I and the Thou.

But the I and the Thou themselves exist on another *pre-ontological* and apophatic level. They are indeed living mysteries to humans. Maybe—as Buber (2013) and Patocka (2015) indicate—the deepest level of wonder is the wonder that emanates from the relation—the in-between—the wonders in and of the I-Thou-relation?

Patocka and Buber call this pre-ontological relation 'love' or a kind of pre-linguistic 'seeing and listening with the heart,' and the wonders that appears in and through this 'in-between-ness' Buber names "*geistige Wesenheiten*" or "spirit in phenomenal forms" (see Wood, 1969, p. 43).

Apophatic or spiritual wonder has to do with being in resonance with the wonder of love and of these 'geistige Wesenheiten' and the mysterious Thou. *Philosophical* wonder has to do with the existential dimension, where the I becomes aware of its own enigmatic nature in relation to the Thou, and the *artistic* wonder might then be some kind of sensuous or soulful wonder, where we through aesthetic means, art works, and practices pave the way to become aware of the lifeworld and Being-dimension that precedes the I-Thou-relation and functions as the gateway to the I-Thou-relation.

If I should relate to the thinking of a scholar in spiritual care, such as Carlo Leget (2017) and his notion of 'inner space' (see chapter 3 in this book) and Harmut Rosa (2019) and the notion of 'resonance,' I would suggest that the 'inner space' can be understood as a two-folded space. The inner space has, as it were, two chambers, a 'welcoming chamber' and a 'heart chamber.' In the first chamber, the person is encouraged to be as open and receptive to all the voices of life and to let them be as they are. This is where we find the relevance of the artistic wonder when it is primary based upon live experiences. In the second chamber, the person relates to the 'goodness' in all these voices, not through reflective discernments and rational choices but through a silent contemplative and heart-listening way. It is in the second chamber that wonder—existential and apophatic wonder—becomes important in terms of hearing the call of both the mysterious Thou and the mysterious I. Who am I in the response to the call of the Thou? What choice do I feel at home within? However, you will also in this chamber be able to find the artistic wonder, when the artwork is primary based on experience of transcendence and sense of mysteries. In this wager, in this saturated silence that follows the deep wonder of all three sorts (the aesthetical, philosophical, and spiritual) a light beyond words shines and makes the heart see. In this kind of deep wonder, we do not look at the world, it is rather the world that look at us, or we now see through the light of the living mysteries of the world. There is an ethics connected to wonder when experienced from within the heart and when seen with the light from the silence that follows wonder. And after silence, that is saturated with wonder, might the inspired or spirited word come.

ETHICS OF WONDER

We can now return to my experience with philosophical practices and Wonder Labs at the Danish hospice and hospital and ask the following: Is it at all possible to '*practice* wonder'? Is deep philosophical wonder—the three forms to which Wittgenstein gave space (transcendental, existential, and the ethical or apophatic wonder)—*not* exactly something that we human beings can construct and control or 'will'? If deep wonder is an ontological event that happens to us and, therefore, bounded to what Harmut Rosa ('Unverfügbarkeit,' Rosa, 2018) describes as the sphere of unavailability, then how do we 'work' with wonder in order to 're-humanize' and 're-enchant' late modern education, health, and welfare?

To answer these questions, I will need to make a distinction between three forms of ethics of wonder: ethics *for* wonder, ethics *of* wonder, and ethics *in the afterglow of* wonder. One could also see these three forms of ethics as the movement of a glider. A glider must have an external force to lift it into the air. When the glider has reached a certain altitude, its buoyancy will carry it on its own. But when the glider has to land, new matters become important, such as a decent landing gear and a runway on the ground. When I facilitate a Wonder Lab, as described at the beginning of this essay, I am like the engine aircraft that forcefully pulls the glider up into the air. What I mainly do is to question, in a Socratic, dialectical, and wondrous way, the participants' rhetorical and tacit taken-for-granted assumptions when they enter the Wonder Lab. During the Wonder Lab, I also train them to ask these Socratic and wondrous questions to themselves. After a while, the 'buoyancy winds of wonder' begin to appear, and when I experience that the participants have now started to philosophize on their own and participate in a community of wonder, I as a facilitator slowly step aside in order for the subject matter, the phenomenon itself, to become the guide of the dialogue. Finally, when the group must end the Wonder Lab and 'land' their wonderments, a new phase emerges. I then help them land their wonderments and new wonder insights in their daily lives and work life. How may these new thoughts and aspirations make a change in their worlds?

I have learned during my many years as a Socratic facilitator that there is an ethics embodied in some Socratic virtues that is important to realize in a Wonder Lab if the participants are to reach the zenith of the curve, that is, the moments when deep wonder takes the lead by itself.

Elsewhere, I have described in depth these seven Socratic virtues (Hansen, 2015, 2018), but briefly said, these are: 1) *love* (to search for or listen to what is the dearest and most precious in one's life, to follow one's passion); 2) *silence* (when listening to what is most precious, you become still and silent, slowly and receiving, in order to hear what the heart, situation/relation calls you to say or think); 3) *humbleness or humility* (when trying to find expressions for the impression from the heart, you notice how small your own words and thoughts are compared to the saturated meaningfulness you feel you are in resonance with; 4) *humour* (looking at one's own life from a grand perspective can sometimes make you feel deep joy and gratefulness because of the beauty and goodness that this light casts on your life and at the same time, makes you laugh because you, with love and mildness, discover how small your own present thinking and living really are when seen in this light. Humour also involves playfulness, imagination, and a feeling of deep spiritual inner freedom, as if your heart was allowed for a short moment to get out of the constrains that normally surround it); 5) *courage* (to be honest and authentic demands that you dare to speak up and put yourself at risk and have the courage to stand in the open without a banister of rules, dogmas or theories); 6) *self-discipline* (having the respect of the discipline and tradition of philosophy and art in order to listen, learn, and try *living* a philosophical life in practice is a demanding self-discipline); and 7) *friendship* (it is a deep joy to find a soul companion that follows you to your own limitations of thought and beyond in search of the better person you aspire to become. The joy is even greater (and respect and playfulness between you and the other) when you are able to meet as companions around something that goes beyond words, but you both seem to long for—or are shaken by. Friendship on this existential ground can, in deep grief or despair, as Patocka (1996, p. 134) so eloquently formulates it, be described as 'a solidarity of the shaken.'

I have experienced that these seven virtues are very important ways of being as a human when one wants to be receptive towards the event of a philosophical wonder and wisdom-seeking dialogues. These virtues help you, so to speak, to look or listen in the right direction. You could also say that these ways of being-in-the-world and being-in-dialogue-with-others nurture an openness and receptiveness that makes you capable of getting into the zone of wonder. By living these virtues, you start thinking and being in dialogue in a much slower and more humble, authentic, caring, and playful way. What you enter as a preparation for deep wonder to occur is, I believe, an 'Inner Space,' which Carlo Leget (2017) so aptly described as an important part of spiritual care.[4] These are virtues of the ethics *for* wonder. This is the ethics where *you* are the agent, to a certain degree, to at least place yourself in the open to be grasped by wonder *if* it arrives.

When it comes to the ethics *of* wonder, one could say that it involves more or less the same virtues but is now experienced in light of being in wonder and experiencing the phenomenon in itself. Therefore, the wonder and phenomenon constitute the agency! This means that the first virtue (*love*) is experienced not as *Eros* (as a desire and longing in the human), but as *Agape* (as a grace and epiphany coming to the human). *Silence* is not an attitude you put yourself into in order to hear better; you are put into silence by something which transcends what you can control and master. *Humbleness* is felt as deep gratitude towards life as such. *Humour* is experienced as if it is life itself that laughs or plays with you. *Courage* is something that you do not decide to be; it is something that the situation/relation calls you to act out. *Self-discipline* is like being an artist when the artist steps aside in order for the materials or colours to shine through or act on or through you. Finally, *friendship* is felt not as a chosen act and attitude but as a spiritual event or embrace that happens to you.

Ethics *in the afterglow of* wonder is when we return to our mundane intentional egos and lives when we are no longer out in the open, taken by wonder, and now try 'to pull the catch in,' which is to learn what the insights of wonder have left in us and what these insights might bring about regarding new ideas for changes and innovation in our daily lives. Here, you may ask, 'Okay, if we want to create a space where wonder may more easily happen to us or to be seen, then what could be practical ethical guidelines to follow in our work culture and life as such?'

WONDER AS A HUMANIZING FORCE: SOME CONCLUDING REMARKS AND SUGGESTED PERSPECTIVES

Let me now end this essay by pointing to two possible consequences of bringing this 'thauma-centric' perspective into current debates on health and education in late modern societies. The first lesson to learn from this perspective is that professionalism and the research on professional relations cannot only be approached from a scientific-empirical and evidence-based approach. This approach is relevant for examining and improving the so-called system- and task-led caring or 'the voice of socialization' and the 'voice of qualification' in education. We also saw that approaching human- or person-centred caring or the 'voice of subjectification' (Biesta, 2010, 2020) only from an existentialistic or social constructivist 'meaning-*making* paradigm' will not be sufficient either. The wonder-based approach and 'thauma-centric worldview' adds some new dimensions to professionalism and research in human and professional relations. First of all, the processes and relations are seen and understood from within a 'meaning-*receiving* paradigm.'

Second, as the figure below shows, what the current theories on 'human- and person-centred caring' and 'voice of being' or 'subjectification' miss is the metaphysical dimension, here described and understood as the sense of wonder or as a *phenomenon- or mystery-led* approach. If we add this metaphysical mystery dimension as a fourth voice or orientation in trying to map the different spheres and dimensions of professional work and knowing and non-knowing, we will also discover four different ways of re-humanizing and re-enchanting the late modern institutions of education, health, and welfare:

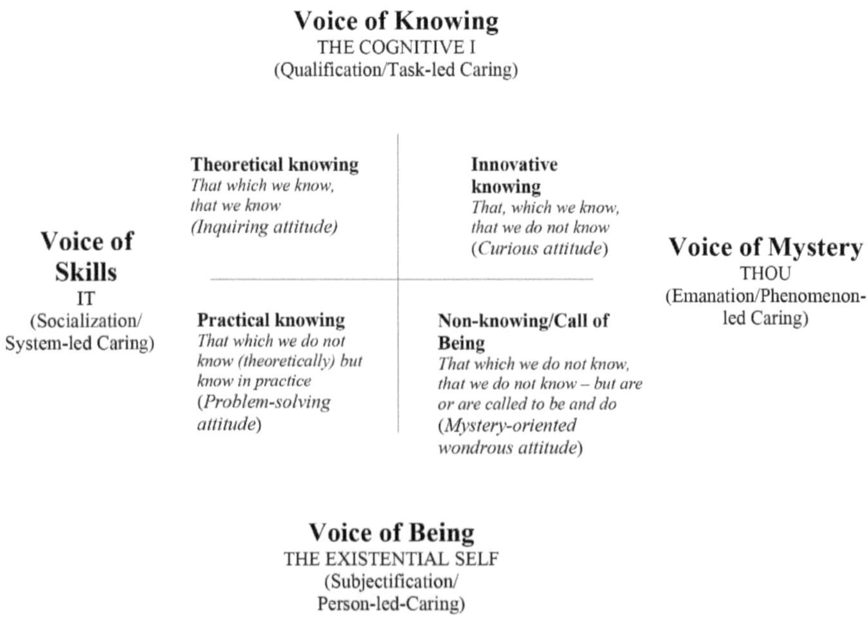

Figure 1.2. Created by Finn Thorbjørn Hansen.

'The trouble of being human these days'—as Zigmunt Bauman phrased it[5]—is, in my view, not only to find ways to balance system- and task-led caring and education with a human- or person-oriented caring and education, as for example the educational philosophers Gert Biesta (2010, 2020) and Ronald Barnett (2007) suggest. This will not fundamentally get us out of an anthropo-centric worldview. The call of transcendence or the Thou, as Patocka and Buber remind us, has a metaphysical and apophatic source. This source, as we have now seen, can be found or revitalized by a growing sense of wonder and sense regarding the mystery in daily life.

Looking at the matrix[6] above, there seem to be three spaces for human flourishing and development that are led by and through knowledge-seeking approaches. The fourth space, however, is of a fundamentally different kind. This space for human flourishing and development is grounded in a fundamental and radical 'non-knowing.' In this space, one will never gain insights or deeper understandings if one arrives solely from within a knowledge-seeking approach. The space opens only if you arrive with a deep sense of wonder. Here, the focus is not on knowing, and in fact, neither is it on Being, as such, because Being is, as it were, only the window through which we must look in order to see or gaze into the living mystery and 'Good beyond Being.'[7]

In Gerd Biesta's research, he talks about 'coming into the world' and 'the arrival of the I' as keys to understanding how we can re-humanize late modern institutions through 'subjectification,' that is, through person-oriented caring and education. What I have argued for in this essay is a fundamentally 'thauma-centric worldview,' which calls for the 'arrival of the mystery.' The I, in an existential sense, always arrives *after* the arrival of the mystery and the wonder that follows. Humans are called to be who they are in their singularity, uniqueness and irreplaceability through wonder. The human and singular person we are, or come to be, is in other words not only due to an encounter with the Other in a Levinasian sense (as a 'radical Other,' which we will never be able to meet). How can we, I wonder, have positive knowledge and certainty, as Levinas seems to have when he talks about the *necessary* asymmetry and superior of the Other? I look at it in another way. In meeting the Other in wonder as a deep, living mystery, and Thou in the Buberian sense, a meeting becomes possible. However, we have no knowledge or understanding whatsoever of how and when this meeting might happen. We can only hope and have faith that, through love and wonder towards the Other or the phenomenon in itself, we *might* experience a meeting and possible union for a short moment, albeit always unexpected as a gift or grace.

The nurses at the Danish hospice and hospital learned to have this reverence for and patience towards the gift of wonder, and they grew into experiences of where and when existential and apophatic wonder was a humanizing force. This gave them trust and faith towards wonder as moments where you can lean into the unknown and meet the other person or live wonders-in-life.

In the following essays in this book, you will see in diverse ways how and why different forms of wonder and silences may call upon different spaces for human flourishing in many different contexts in education, health care and welfare.

NOTES

1. By 'apophatic,' I refer to the philosophical reception of the tradition of 'negative theology,' which focuses on 'unsayable,' enigmatic but deeply meaningful phenomena in our lifeworld, only approachable from a kind of 'negative ontology' or 'negative metaphysics' or 'anatheism' (Cooper, 2002; Franke, 2014; Kearney, 2011, 2016; Rhodes, 2012).

2. The relationship between Wittgenstein's philosophy and the I-Thou-philosophy of the two philosophers of dialogue, Rosenzweig and Buber, is described in Putnam (2008).

3. It is key to the understanding of existential phenomenology that one can make a distinction between 'the ontic' and 'the ontological' dimensions of life and work. In the 'ontic' worldview, human beings are in control and see the world and the things they do as something functional to be and mastered. The pragmatic and common sense, as well as the scientific attitude and work approach, are part of the ontic worldview. Regarding the 'ontological' worldview, in the Heideggerian sense, you are always already a 'being-in-the-world' before you reflect on it, have intentions with it or act to control it. The ontological sense or awareness is a sense of being very present in the world, as a moment when being carries you or speaks to you, like a painter might say that a tree he is painting is 'speaking back' to him in the process of artistic creation.

4. For a description of the relation between 'the inner space' and wonder and Wonder Labs, please see Leget's chapter in this anthology.

5. https://vimeo.com/ondemand/beinghuman.

6. I first presented this matrix in another context where the relationship between philosophical wonder and innovation in higher education was the issue (Hansen, 2020b).

7. See also Allen (2009).

REFERENCES

Allen, S. (2009). *The Philosophical Sense of Transcendence: Levinas and Plato on Loving Beyond Being*. Pittsburg: Duquesne University Press.

Arendt, H. (2018). *Thinking Without a Banister*. New York: Penguin Random House.

Barnett, R. (2007). *A Will to Learn: Being a Student in an Age of Uncertainty*. London: Open University Press.

Beale, J. & Kidd, I. (eds.) (2017). *Wittgenstein and Scientism*. London: Routledge.

Biesta, G. (2010). *Good Education in an Age of Measurement: Ethics, Politics*. Boulder, CO: Paradigm Publishers.

Biesta, G. (2020). Risking ourselves in education: qualification, socialization, and subjectification revisited. *Educational Theory*, Vol. 70(1): 89–104.

Bortoft, H. (2012). *Taking Appearance Seriously: The Dynamic Way of Seeing in Goethe and European Thought*. Edinburgh: Floris Books.

Buber, M. (1970/1923). *I and Thou*. Translated by Walter Kaufmann. New York: Scribner.

Buber, M. (2013/1923). *I and Thou*. Translated by Ronald Gregor Smith. London: Bloomsbury Academic.

Cooper, D. (2002). *The Measure of Things: Humanism, Humility, and Mystery*. Oxford: Clarendon Press.

Cooper, D. (2018). *Senses of Mystery*. New York: Routledge.

Dreyfus, H. & Kelly, S.D. (2011). *All Things Shinning: Reading the Western Classics to Find Meaning in a Secular Age*. New York: Free Press.

Franke, W. (2014). *A Philosophy of the Unsayable*. Notre Dame, IN: University of Notre Dame Press.

Galvin, K. & Todres, L. (2013). *Caring and Well-being: A Lifeworld Approach*. London: Routledge.

Hadot, P. (1995). *Philosophy as a Way of Life: Spiritual Exercises from Socrates to Foucault*. Oxford: Blackwell Publishing.

Hadot, P. (2002). *What Is Ancient Philosophy?* Cambridge, Mass.: Harvard University Press.

Hansen, F.T. (2010). *At stå I det åbne. Dannelse gennem filosofisk undren og nærvær* [To Stand in the Openness: Bildung through Philosophical Wonder and Presence]. Copenhagen: Hans Reitzel.

Hansen, F.T. (2013). *Filosofisk vejledning og praktisk kundskab på professionsuddannelser* [Philosophical Counseling and Practical Knowledge in Human-related Professions]. Research report. University of Aalborg, Open Access: https://vbn.aau.dk/da/publications/filosofisk-vejledning-og-praktisk-kundskab-på-professionsuddannel.

Hansen, F.T. (2014). *Kan man undre sig uden ord? Design- og universitetspædagogik på kreative videregående uddannelser* [Can One Wonder Without Words? Design and University Pedagogy on Creative Higher Educations]. Aalborg: Aalborg Universitetsforlag.

Hansen, F.T. (2015). The call and practice of wonder: how to evoke a Socratic community of wonder in professional settings. In: Noah Weiss, M. (ed.), *Socratic Handbook: Dialogue Methods for Philosophical Practice* (s. 217–244). Wien: LIT Verlag.

Hansen, F.T. (2016). *At undre sig ved livets afslutning: Om brug af filosofiske samtaler i palliativt arbejde* [To Wonder at the End of Life: On the Use of Philosophical Conversations in Palliative Care]. Copenhagen: Akademisk forlag.

Hansen, F.T. (2018). *At møde verden med undren: Dannelse, innovation og organisatorisk udvikling i et værensfilosofisk perspektiv* [To Encounter the World Through Wonder: Bildung, Innovation and Organizational Development in an Existential Perspective]. Copenhagen: Hans Reitzel.

Hansen, F.T. (2020a). Professionel kontakt handler også om at være i takt med det underfulde [Professional contact is also about being intact with the wonderful]. In: Alrø, H., Billund, L. & Herholdt-Lomholdt, S. (eds.), *Professionel kontakt* (pp. 101–120). Aalborg: Aalborg Universitetsforlag.

Hansen, F.T. (2020b). Learning to innovate in higher education through deep wonder. *Philosophy and Theory in Higher Education.* Vol. 1(3): pp. 51–74.

Hansen, F.T. & Jørgensen, L. (2020). A contribution to the ontology of the fundamentals of care framework from a wonder-based approach. *Journal of Clinical Nursing*, Vol. X: pp. 1797–1807. https://doi.org/10.1111/jocn.15272.

Heidegger, M. (1962). *Being and Time*. Trans. John Macquarrie and Edward Robinson. San Francisco: Harper.

Heschel, A. (1965). *Who Is Man?* Stanford: Stanford University Press.

Kleiman, S. (2009). *Human Centered Nursing: The Foundation of Quality Care*. Philadelphia: F.A. Davis.

Leget, C. (2017). *Art of Living, Art of Dying: Spiritual Care for Good Death*. London: Jessica Kingsley Publishers.

Martinsen, K. (2018). *Bevegelig Berørt* [Movingly Touched]. Bergen: Fakbokforlaget.

McCormack, B. & McCance, T. (2017). *Person-centred Practice in Nursing and Health Care: Theory and Practice*. Oxford: Wiley Blackwell.

Patocka, J. (1989). Negative Platonism: reflections concerning the rise, the scope, and the demise of metaphysics—and whether philosophy can survive it. In: Kohák, E. (ed), *Jan Patocka: Philosophy and Selected Writings* (pp. 175–206). Chicago: The University of Chicago Press.

Patocka, J. (1996). *Heretical Essays in the Philosophy of History*. Chicago: Open Court.

Patocka, J. (2002). *Plato and Europe*. Stanford: Stanford University Press.

Patocka, J. (2015/1977). On Masaryk's philosophy of religion. In: Hagedorn, L. & Dodd, J. (eds.), *The New Yearbook for Phenomenology and Phenomenological Philosophy*, Vol. XIV (A special issue dedicated to the philosophy of Jan Patocka (pp. 95–135). London: Routledge.

Putnam, H. (2008). *Jewish Philosophy as a Guide to Life: Rosenzweig, Buber, Levinas, Wittgenstein*. Bloomington: Indiana University Press.

Rhodes, M. (2012). *Mystery in Philosophy: An Invocation of Pseudo-Dionysius*. Lanham: Lexington Books.

Rosa, H. (2018). *Unverfügbarkeit*. Wien: Residenz Verlag.

Shusterman, R. (1997). *Practicing Philosophy: Pragmatism and the Philosophical Life*. New York: Routledge.

Sugarman, R. (2002). Emmanuel Levinas: The ethics of 'face to face'/religious turn. In: Tymieniecka, A.T. (ed.), *Phenomenology World Wide* (pp. 409–459). London: Kluwer Academic Publishers.

Taylor, C. (2007). *A Secular Age*. Cambridge, MA: Harvard University Press.

Visse, M. (2012). *Openings for Humanization in Modern Health Care Practices* (PhD-dissertation), the University of VRIJE, the Netherlands: https://www.researchgate.net/publication/301285269_Openings_for_humanization_in_modern_health_care_practices

Wittgenstein, L. (1965). Lectures on ethics. *The Philosophical Review*, Vol. 74(1): 3–12.

Wittgenstein, L. (1969). *On Certainty*. Oxford: Basil Blackwell.

Wittgenstein, L. (1998). *Culture and Value* (revised ed.). Oxford: Blackwell Publishing.

Chapter 2

Inner Space, Resonance, and Wonder

The Humanization of Health Care in Small Steps

Carlo Leget

A 24-year-old psychologist was lying in the hospital waiting to hear about the nature of her medical condition. She had gone to her general practitioner after noticing strange pulsating motions in the right half of her face: the doctor had been unable to diagnose her but suspected neurological problems such as migraine or a minor stroke. She was admitted to the hospital and underwent a week of medical examinations: a week full of worry, uncertainty, and disbelief.

When after a week the neurologist entered the room, she communicated the news quickly and effectively: 'You have multiple sclerosis.' The young woman was shocked, and the first question that came to her mind was: 'Is this a chronic condition?' The neurologist answered: 'Yes, it is.' Understanding the nature of her condition and its possible genetic implications, the patient asked: 'Can I still have children?' The neurologist laughed, and responded, 'Well, multiple sclerosis has nothing to do with your ovaries.' As the patient started to cry, the neurologist turned her back on her, and said: 'You're a psychologist, so you know how to deal with this.' Then she tapped on the patient's lower legs and left the room.

When we reflect on the humanization of health care, it is sometimes helpful to start with real-life examples that give food for thought. Whatever our conception of humanization, we would probably agree that this is not an instance of humane interaction in a health care setting. The neurologist never visited the patient again, which is difficult to understand from a professional point of view. Nevertheless, it is a small everyday example of what happens in hospitals in northwest Europe and probably all over the globe.

Incidents like these have no witnesses apart from the two or three people involved, and almost never result in formal complaints. We do not know how often they happen, but we do know that they have a huge impact on patients. More than ten years later, the woman still has tears in her eyes when she tells the story: she was deeply hurt that day, and the pain is still there like an injury that starts to burn immediately as it is touched.

In this contribution, I will focus on the humanization of health care practices by discussing something that is present in humane interactions, but almost never addressed as such: a quality that I call 'inner space.' This metaphor seeks to express something that I consider of great importance for living a good life. Inner space is something we all know from experience, and it connects everyday human encounters with bigger cultural and societal questions about the world we live in.

I will begin by sketching the discovery of inner space in my earlier work. Then I will connect these reflections with the work of Hartmut Rosa and Finn Hansen, to show how inner space may contribute to what I consider to be the core of humanization: being in resonance with the world and the people around us, and their 'speaking' to us in a way that is as transformative for us as it is to them.

THE INVENTION OF 'INNER SPACE'

I opened this chapter with a short story from a hospital, setting the stage with an example of what humanization is not. Because this is far from exceptional, many authors in recent decades have discussed how we can reform the health care sector to prevent such situations.

One way of approaching this question is by focusing on the system. We have organized health care in such a way that highly paid medical specialists must work under enormous time pressure. Moreover, medical students are selected for their brains, and not for their hearts. And it is well documented that empathy declines during medical education, especially when interns start to become socialized by bad role models. Where problems are framed this way, and they should be, it is possible to start looking for solutions. Sometimes health care professionals are trained to become more empathic and compassionate, and there has been an increasing investment in medical humanities over recent years.

One of the specific ways humanization has been promoted is through the development of spiritual care (Cobb, Puchalski, & Rumbold, 2012). This can be defined as an interdisciplinary approach to the existential dimension of health care. The word 'existential' in this chapter refers to the search for the meaning of one's existence and the role of connectedness in this, rather than to existentialism as a philosophical or psychological tradition. Spiritual care involves givers and receivers and may be religious or non-religious. It is a common responsibility of all health care professionals and volunteers, leading to a variety of shared practices.

The development of spiritual care over the last few decades is an important move towards the humanization of health care, bringing back a dimension of meaning that had sometimes been lost when focusing too much on the physical and psychosocial dimensions. It is the movement that comes closest to paying attention to the healing dimension of health care, restoring the resonance with inspiration from beyond that which we initiate or control ourselves, and opening towards the transformative dimension of suffering.

What criteria should we use in identifying good spiritual care? Broadly speaking, authors have sought to answer this question in two ways. Some have adopted the standards of specific religious or secular traditions. In Roman Catholicism for example, good spiritual care is about being at peace with oneself, one's neighbors, and God. In the end, only God can decide whether someone is really at peace in these three relationships, although Catholics are assured that there are good reasons to be confident that they are on the right path when they follow the wisdom of their tradition.

Other authors try to build spiritual care on a secular and non-denominational basis. Their criterion is whether care meets the needs of patients and families who ask for it. These two types of answers can be in tension with each other, because what a religious tradition asks from a patient (such as forgiveness and reconciliation) may differ from patients' and families' expressed needs, such as recognition and justice. In this contribution, I will focus on secular spiritual care.

Based on the implicit needs of the young woman described at the beginning of the chapter, the neurologist has failed to provide good spiritual care in several ways. In the first place, her communication showed a general lack of decency and humaneness. Her behavior was not attuned to the patient's emotional state, her reference to the patient's profession was inappropriate, her response to the patient's question was insulting, and she did not end the conversation properly or provide any form of aftercare. In fact, one might ask whether this was a human conversation at all. There was no connection between the two people involved: one simply dumped sensitive information on the other in a way that, from a moral perspective, was almost an act of violence. In the second place, the neurologist failed to address the existential dimension of the situation. Telling a young woman that she has a serious chronic condition that will affect every dimension of her life means taking part in someone else's life event. This brings great responsibilities.

In the last twenty years I have introduced a new dimension to palliative spiritual care based on the late medieval *ars moriendi,* the art of dying (Leget, 2007; 2016; 2017). This tradition took the form of small, illustrated booklets on how to prepare for a good death, which appeared after the spread of bubonic plague in Europe between 1346 and 1353. They were written for patients, not caregivers, and were organized around five great temptations at the end of life, covering important virtues like hope, faith, charity, patience, and humility. In my retrieval of this tradition, I rephrased the five temptations into five struggles in which patients are torn between two opposite poles, such as self/other, doing/undergoing, holding on/letting go, remembering/forgetting, and knowing/believing. This contemporary *ars moriendi* was developed as a conversation model for patients, relatives, and caregivers, aimed at dealing with the many existential challenges that may come up at the end of life. Although it is primarily written for patients, dying is seen as a social process in which all participants have a great impact on one another.

The criterion for a good death in the late medieval art of dying was being accepted by God and admitted to heaven. In the contemporary version, I replaced this with the metaphor of 'inner space,' putting more emphasis on the quality of the process and social interactions than a metaphysical outcome. Inner space is a metaphor for several lived experiences. It can refer to attentiveness in an open and non-judgmental manner that is not directed towards a specific object and manifests itself as a basic mood (*Grundstimmung*) that colors one's lived experiences. It may also refer to having thoughts, emotions, feelings, or moods and simultaneously being aware of these phenomena without being determined or dominated by them. So inner space is not a synonym for what is sometimes called the soul, as the place or faculty of spiritual processes. It is an aspect of freedom within spiritual, cognitive, and emotional processes.

One of the reasons why I chose inner space as a central metaphor was because I wanted to find a phrase expressing what seemed to be the distinctive quality of the way I saw people listening, speaking, communicating, and being with one another. When they did this in a good and supportive way, there seemed to be gentleness, connectedness, humor, and room for exchange based on confidence. This quality is not static but may change its appearance and modality. The more inner space I perceived in people, the better the quality of their communication and interaction seemed to be; in fact, in my experience the quality of inner space was often transmitted from one person to another. Just as a good or bad mood can be transmitted nonverbally, people with inner space can help others to develop it themselves. By staying close to the real struggles of a process as existential as dying, the metaphor of inner space helped me to avoid overly idealistic aspirations in end-of-life care, such as the ideal of inner peace that may make patients and families feel they have failed if they have not reached it.

The 'art of dying' model has been well received in my country and has clearly helped many people seeking direction at a difficult time of life. It helped them to seek their unique way of dealing with five big existential questions that may come up at the end of life: Who am I and what do I really want? How do I deal with suffering? How can I say goodbye? How do I look back on my life? What can I hope for? The contemporary conversation model situates these questions in the framework of five polarities that do not represent a good and a bad side or answer but are general anthropological categories that are in tension with each other.

One aspect that was an eye-opener to some, and greatly appreciated by others, was that the metaphor of inner space helps us to acknowledge and even appreciate the tensions and conflicting thoughts, emotions, feelings, and moods that we may experience. As long as there is inner space, it may be fruitful to listen to thoughts and feelings, since they can all tell us something worth hearing. It liberates us from an internalized moral viewpoint distinguishing between good and bad feelings. It is like listening to an inner polyphony, a choir in which we can hear individual voices and the harmonic or dissonant whole they form. If we listen to it without inner space, we may be completely absorbed by some of the voices or the whole choir. The cacophony or harmony may be so compelling or overwhelming that they take away our inner space, and with it the freedom of subjectivity.

In this contribution, I will seek to explain how inner space can help when reflecting on the humanization of health care. I will do this by engaging in dialogue with the work of the German sociologist Hartmut Rosa, and the Danish philosopher Finn Thorbjørn Hansen. Working from different traditions and paradigms, both scholars help to articulate what the contribution of inner space may be. I will first present Hartmut Rosa's concept of resonance and reflect on how this can help further to develop the idea of inner space. Then I will turn to Finn Hansen's work on wonder and ask whether his phenomenological approach implies something like inner space, and how it can contribute to the humanization of health care.

RESONANCE

In 2016, Hartmut Rosa published a book later translated as *Resonance. A sociology of our relationship to the world* (Rosa, 2016). The book is the fruit of more than twenty years' research and reflection on the crisis of the present age, which he diagnoses as a crisis of acceleration. Contemporary developments are built on noble intentions: to humanize life and increase our freedom by making the world more 'available' through countless scientific and technological developments. Making the world available, in Rosa's view, has four elements: making it visible, accessible, controllable, and usable (Rosa, 2019, pp. 21–24).

Although many people undeniably enjoy a longer life expectancy and higher economic standards than ever before in history, something fundamental seems to have happened with our relationship to the world. Our economic system is built on an imperative of escalating growth that can be stabilized only by continuous economic expansion, technological acceleration, and cultural innovation. This imperative enforces the dominance of a reifying relationship with the world in which even our leisure time is commodified and exploited. As a result, the world has gradually been made 'mute': things do not 'speak' to us anymore but are reduced to dead material that can be used, manipulated, or even exploited to enlarge our chances of happiness or wellbeing.

How such a 'muting' of the world may work out in medical practice is well illustrated by the narrative at the beginning of this contribution. The patient does not 'speak' to the neurologist in the sense of being seen as a unique, vulnerable, and dependent human being. So, she is almost literally muted: the neurologist dumps information on her, laughs at an existential question, and turns her back on the patient.

In his book, Rosa develops an answer to the alienation that has become characteristic of our relationship to the world, by introducing the concept of resonance. In his own words:

> Resonance is a kind of relationship to the world, formed through af←fect and e→motion, intrinsic interest, and perceived self-efficacy, in which subject and world are mutually affected and transformed.
>
> Resonance is not an echo, but a responsive relationship, requiring that both sides speak *with their own voice.* This is only possible where strong evaluations are affected. Resonance implies an aspect of constitutive inaccessibility *[Unverfügbarkeit].*
>
> Resonant relationships require that both subject and world be sufficiently "closed" or self-consistent so as to each speak in their own voice, while also remaining open enough to be affected or reached by each other.
>
> Resonance is not an emotional state, but a mode of relation that is neutral with respect to emotional content. This is why we can love sad stories. (Rosa, 2016, p. 174)

When we think of the humanization of health care, welfare, and education, Rosa's work on resonance offers an analysis and conceptualization that is helpful in addressing our contemporary crises. Where most publications on spiritual care focus on the relationship between meaning and connectedness on a personal, interpersonal or institutional level, his approach is rooted in a critical analysis of contemporary society that lays bare the foundations of our situation. From this perspective, it is possible critically to reflect on the way spiritual care is introduced and used to humanize health care.

In the first place, spiritual care as an interdisciplinary field of study has many tensions in itself. On the one hand, it is largely inspired by religious traditions that are very much aware of the inaccessibility and unavailability of the mystery at their center. On the other hand, to be compatible with and acceptable to the world of health care, they use a logic of scientific rigor (causality and predictability) that is contrary to the very core of spirituality and religion (Leget, 2020). Rosa's work makes us question whether spiritual care risks losing its original intuition of a reality beyond what we can think and speak of.

Secondly, the concept of resonance brings in a new language to conceptualize and reflect on what the literature on spiritual care speaks of mainly in terms of purpose, goal, meaning, and connectedness (Puchalski et al., 2014). Where these concepts are easily integrated in psychological categories and scientific approaches compatible with mainstream health care research, spiritual care runs the risk of being directed at spiritual coping in one way or another. In this coping approach, spirituality is seen instrumentally, as a psychological mechanism that helps to deal with a situation.

As a contrast to this psychological framework, Rosa's approach opens an alternative means of access to the existential dimension by focusing on a mode of relationship with the world in which respect for otherness, unavailability, and transformation play a central role. These three elements are constitutive of a responsive relationship, and this is precisely what lies at the core of humanization.

If we think again of the neurologist at the beginning of this chapter, we see the opposite of a responsive relationship. There is an object relation between physician and patient, a refusal to be affected or transformed by the other person, and a denial of unavailability. The message is dumped without any interest in how it is received. What could have been a transformative encounter, in which the patient was supported in her existential fears and questions, building a life-sustaining web between physician and patient, was in fact an act of dehumanization and abandonment (Tronto, 1993).

If we now turn back to the metaphor of inner space, as the core of the *ars moriendi* conversation model designed to open towards the existential dimension of life, and as a way to become aware of the polyphony inside oneself, how does this relate to Rosa's theory of resonance?

As I see it, in the *ars moriendi* model, inner space can play a double role as both the seed and the fruit of spiritual processes. It can work as a precondition to be open to the polyphony of voices and possible dissonance that may be involved. At the same time, inner space can be the result of a process in which these inner voices have been heard and recognized. But the metaphor does not describe how the many voices may play a role in spiritual processes. Here, the concept of resonance may be helpful. Inner space can be seen as the aspect of freedom inherent in open and non-judgmental awareness of experiences of resonance and alienation or even repulsion. The difference between inner space and mindfulness is that inner space is not an attitude of open indifference and dissociation between cognition, emotions, and feelings on the one hand, and reality on the other. In my view its importance is that it enables us to 'hold' the mixture of positive and negative cognition and emotions to investigate what this mixture has to tell us. Using the vocabulary of resonance, one could also say that inner space allows the responsive relationship of resonance to take place and the transformation to be experienced.

Interestingly, like resonance, inner space is not an emotional state, but a mode of relation that is neutral with respect to emotional content. Like resonance, it is open to dissonance, and to respecting otherness. What resonance adds to inner space is pointing to the transformative aspect of the experience that is part of a truly responsive relationship. Where inner space helps to remain open towards receiving and respecting otherness, like a kind of hospitality that avoids both annexation and othering, it can be a precondition for transformative experiences by which otherness becomes a source of development and growth. Listening with inner space, the neurologist would not have reduced the unknown young woman to the category of patients with MS (annexation and othering) but could have resonated with the existential dimension of her new situation and the questions it provoked. At the same time, inner space can never be a guarantee of resonance: the aspect of unavailability inherent in resonance inhibits any control of this phenomenon.

But what does this mean for the normativity of inner space and resonance? If we reflect on the role of spirituality in the humanization of health care, we might ask whether every transformation is a good transformation. How can we discern between good and bad? For example, could we consider the experience of the woman in our narrative as a transformative experience of negative resonance that might build up a more resilient attitude towards physicians?

At the end of his book, Hartmut Rosa rejects the idea of negative resonance, acknowledging that this idea is one of the most difficult conceptual problems of his theory. I believe that the answer to this question depends on the way one conceptualizes good and bad and distinguishes between them. Rosa develops his theory of resonance as an answer to the phenomenon of alienation, which is negative because it signifies a relationship of indifference or hostility to the world: one of repulsion. In Rosa's view, in a state of alienation, the world cannot be adaptively transformed, and can therefore be called non-responsive: a relationship of relationlessness (Rosa, 2016, p. 184).

If we apply this to the dehumanizing situation we described, one could say that the neurologist's relationship to the world is one of alienation. But what about the patient? Does the fact that she is hurt by the incident not indicate that she has been affected and transformed, in the sense that her original state of openness and integrity is wounded and possibly transformed into a situation of alertness and carefulness towards physicians? Is perversion in the end not also a form of transformation with possibly positive aspects?

Rosa would probably respond that if we analyze the woman's situation after the incident, her ability to develop a resonant relationship to the world is diminished rather than enlarged. This means that her ability to experience transformative positive experiences, helping her to develop further as a human being, is reduced, because she will be inclined to close herself off from the risk of being hurt again. By turning away from the world, or taking a stance of indifference, she is defending herself against repeated hurt. In this case, she has tears in her eyes more than ten years after the incident, it resulted in a trauma that risked depriving her of humaneness rather than developing it.

Now that we have seen how the concepts of inner space and resonance can help to analyze dehumanizing moments in health care, could it also be helpful to imagine a more humanizing encounter between the neurologist and her patient? The story at the beginning of this article is told from a third-person perspective. We do not have any insight into the lived experience of the two parties to the conversation, but on superficial examination neither neurologist nor patient seems to display any signs of inner space. The patient's two questions (Is it a chronic condition, and can I still have children?) may seem factual but asked in this specific context it is clear that they are fueled by fear and panic. The questions seem to pop up immediately as her most urgent priorities in getting a grip on this new situation. She asks both with the hope that the answer will be a reassuring no, against all odds. If the neurologist had inner space, this dimension of fear and panic might have resonated, and she might have sensed the existential dimension of the two questions. Inner space would have made her sense that the factual questions concealed existential issues that asked for empathy and comfort.

So, the first important role inner space can play in the encounter between neurologist and patient is to give space to the processes the patient is going through. Humanization of health care can be seen as restoring her as a human being, a moral actor with sufficient inner freedom to make independent choices. Secondly, it could mean giving her space to discover the meaning of what is happening and interpret it within the larger context of her life. Both questions are about the future, about human flourishing, about hope. Neither answer fosters the patient's inner space and freedom, nor helps to develop a future in which she can flourish.

A humanizing encounter between the neurologist and the patient would be sensitive and open to the existential depth of the situation from the patient's perspective. It would start by giving space to what is behind the factual questions. Giving space begins with a quality of inner space, which enables 'hospitality' towards the patient's anxiety that is acknowledged instead of being denied or neglected. Next to a physical place, a hospital is also a spiritual place requiring hospitality to patients' spiritual suffering (Sulmasy, 2006). This enables an encounter of mutual resonance that may be transformative and changes both the 'host' and the 'guest.'

A transformative encounter requires inner space that enables the professional to open up and attune herself to the patient, and inner space in the patient that helps her to experience a wider horizon than that blocked by fears. Thus, keeping space open in communication is dependent on certain qualities in those who communicate. Next to inner space, one of these is an awareness of the weight of words. As Hans Georg Gadamer has brilliantly explained in his work *Truth and method*, language and thought are intimately connected, and since language is the medium through which we are able to share thoughts, its sensitive and responsible use is of utmost importance for humane communication in delicate circumstances. How this works is very well displayed in a recent novel by the philosopher and author Pascal Mercier.

THE WEIGHT OF WORDS

In *Das Gewicht der Worte* (The weight of words), Mercier tells the story of Simon Leyland, an English translator in his early sixties who lives in Trieste and is suddenly diagnosed with a brain tumor and given no more than a year to live (Mercier, 2020). The novel can be read as a sophisticated meditation on the role of words in our lives. As readers, we become more and more sensitive to the value (weight) of words in giving access to the world we live in. We live in words, and every language offers a particular access to reality. Sharing the inner world of the main character in his work as a translator, we experience how precisely this art works, and how translating a sentence is first 'living' it and then rephrase it.

In one of the most beautiful pages in the book, one of Leyland's former colleagues tells him that he recently visited a church and saw a woman cleaning and restoring an old mosaic (Mercier, 2020, pp. 360–61). She was completely absorbed in her work with brushes and spatula and did not care how long it would take or whether anyone would see the result. The only thing that mattered was that the stones in the mosaic would shine again afterwards. The man envied her ability to live in the present moment. Reflecting on this, Leyland realizes that poetry in the broad sense (including visual arts and music) is related to time in that it helps us to let go of past and future and be in the present. We are not just touched by poetry but lifted in a way that makes us more connected with ourselves and puts us in a different relationship with the world.

As a contrast to Simon Leyland's sensitive and respectful awareness of the weight of words, the novel critically reflects on their role in medicine and law. In both sectors, they—and referring to their professional clothes Leyland speaks of the white (medicine) and the black (law) caste—words are used to decide between life and death.

We have already seen the impact of a few words from a physician. In Leyland's case, the diagnosis makes his world fall apart. He decides to sell the publishing house he has inherited from his wife and managed for the past nine years. After seventy-seven days, however, it turns out that his diagnosis is based on medical sloppiness: someone at the hospital had put another patient's brain scan in an envelope with Leyland's name on it, and the physician has failed to check the small words at the margins of the brain scan with the name of the patient. After selling the company and moving to London, Leyland suddenly hears of the mistake. The weight of words, in this case a false diagnosis, can be damaging, especially when these words bear no relation to reality.

The novel also discusses a similar problem in the domain of law. Various characters are personally or professionally involved in cases where people have been convicted for killing others. But each of these is constructed according to a legal logic that does not do justice to reality. In one case, a man puts his heart and soul into taking care of his sick wife for ten years, day and night. She suffers terribly, and repeatedly asks him to end her misery. Eventually he commits a mercy killing and is jailed for murder. He gets the same sentence as another character who comes home unexpectedly, catches his wife with her lover, and kills the lover.

The weight of words in medicine and law is great: a diagnosis and a sentence make the difference between life and death, shape lives, open or close down futures, and can bring both great suffering and great relief. But there is another similarity between medicine and law: words may create and become a reality on their own, separated from what they were supposed to express. The weight of words can be so great that, even when they are separated from the health or justice they are supposed to serve, their power can destroy lives.

Therefore, Leyland demands from every single physician and judge the same acuteness, sensitivity and patience that he displays as a good and conscientious translator. The weight of words is too great to treat lightheartedly.

Leyland is very clear about what he considers to be the major problem with medicine and law: both bear an enormous responsibility connected to the weight of words but have become arrogant and elitist. They distance themselves even further from the vulnerable people they earn their incomes from by cloaking everything in pseudolanguage, a mixture of borrowed Latin and Greek words. Using dead languages to create social distance is symbolic: it expresses what happens when words are used without being connected to lived reality and experiences.

Pascal Mercier's novel resonates strongly with the story of the woman with multiple sclerosis. Because words structure our thinking, speaking, and actions, and can humanize or dehumanize health care, perhaps we do need something else next to inner space and resonance that helps us to open towards what lies beyond words. For this, we will turn to phenomenology and the work of Danish philosopher Finn Thorbjørn Hansen.

PHENOMENOLOGY AND WONDER

One of the great merits of phenomenological research is that it opens new ways of looking at things we thought we already knew. There are many reasons why this can be valuable. In the encounter between the neurologist and the patient, it is obvious that a new way of looking at (and subsequently experiencing) a hopeless situation would be a great consolation for the patient.

A cynic might argue that all this may be true, but that the woman asked for factual information, and that is precisely what she got, communicated clearly and directly in such a way that it was unlikely to be forgotten. We should not spiritualize everything. But we have seen that the patient was still in tears more than ten years after the diagnosis, showing that sometimes asking for facts is not what it seems to be. Inner space could help the neurologist to be sensitive to layers of meaning other than the factual; it could help the patient to discover that there is more than anxiety going on in herself. It could enable processes of resonance that would bring new inspiration and perspective into her life.

The philosopher Havi Carel, who was herself diagnosed with a lung condition in 2006, has written a philosophical analysis of the experience of illness, based on phenomenology (Carel, 2014). She later developed a phenomenological toolkit for patients (Carel, 2012). What triggered her work was the experience that the objective, naturalistic approach to illness, excluding first-person experience, does not help people to live with it. There has been little philosophical analysis of illness, though its impact on all domains of life is considerable.

The first step in Carel's toolkit involves inviting the patient to see illness as a form of phenomenological reduction: a suspension of the 'natural attitude' towards illness to reconstruct their first-person experience. With this impressively simple move, Carel builds a bridge between illness and phenomenology. Going further into her work and toolkit is not the aim of this contribution, as helpful as it might be. Let us, with Carel's invitation in mind, turn back to the young woman in the story at the beginning of this contribution. The neurologist entered the room and communicated the news quickly and effectively: 'You have multiple sclerosis.' Remembering the weight of words, it is not surprising that the patient was shocked. She had been labeled with a relatively well-known disease evoking associations with wheelchairs—a horror scenario for a sporty young woman who had run a marathon two years before. As her two questions were answered and laughed at, and she was basically told to sort out the problem herself, her response was a complete inner disconnection from the diagnosis. Although multiple sclerosis patients are recommended to start medication immediately, she left the hospital and did not talk to a physician again until her first attack one year later.

Now consider an alternative scenario. The neurologist comes in, takes a seat, meets the eyes of the young woman, and asks: 'How are you today?' She listens to her experiences and says something like this: 'I've studied the results of the tests we did this week, and we're pretty sure about what seems to be going on in your body. Your immune system is attacking the myelin, the protective sheath that covers your nerve fibers, and causing communication problems between your brain and the rest of your body. We estimate that there are around 125,000 people in this country who have the same problem. It's different in every individual case, and we don't know what yours will look like. Therefore some people call it the disease of a thousand faces. We don't have a medication that can cure it yet, but we can help to suppress the attacks, like the one that brought you to the hospital this time. There are lots of people who manage fine with it, and we'll do our best to make your life as good as possible.'

We do not know what the patient's response would have been, but this alternative scenario would give her a completely different entry to the world of chronic illness. One of her first questions would probably have been: 'But what kind of disease do I have?' or 'Is it MS?' This is very likely, because this is the way we are socialized in health care as professional caregivers and patients. By following this alternative scenario, however, the communication is completely different. It starts with connecting to the patient, both physically and emotionally, and the neurologist displays a maximum of openness and perspective, without beating around the bush or being vague. The message as regards the physical process and the statistics is very precise, but there is openness and hope as to how the condition will affect this unique patient and what the future will look like. In other words, it is breaking bad news without breaking the patient.

The alternative scenario is a way to communicate a difficult message while attempting to preserve and respect the patient's inner space as much as possible. By doing this, she may be able to live with a chronic disease while enjoying a fulfilled life. This scenario offers possibilities of resonance that were blocked completely in the real-life event.

A lot more will have to be done, from the diagnosis onwards, if health care is to become humanized. In the last few decades, spiritual care has been used as an approach to support patients and their families in the existential dimension of their situation. But to what extent does it help to foster inner space, promote resonance, and keep patients in touch with the phenomenon of life in its inexhaustible richness and power of renewal? How can we develop such an approach, respecting the aspect of unavailability typical of the transformative processes inherent in resonance?

WONDER LABS—A WAY TO GO?

One of the most fascinating examples of this approach are the Wonder Labs, developed by Finn Thorbjørn Hansen (2020). Combining Max van Manen's phenomenology with Steen Halling's dialogical approach, Hansen has worked on the transformative power of wonder as a new access to phenomena.

Wonder (as opposed to curiosity) is characterized by being fascinated in a non-instrumental way. It happens and cannot be planned. There is always an element of unavailability to it, which is connected to its creative nature. The creative aspect of wonder is in turn connected to the phenomenon of speaking, and opens the possibility of resonance, including a transformative process. Wonder Labs are virtual spaces where former experiences of wonder are investigated, and its transformative potential is nurtured by bringing it into resonance with the experiences of other Wonder Labs participants and with great works of art (Hansen, 2015). But how could a Wonder Lab work in the case of the woman diagnosed with MS? How could this benefit her as a form of spiritual care, if she were prepared to participate?

As Wonder Labs start with an experience of wonder, the first question would be whether she can remember an event in which she felt this emotion in relation to her illness. She might recall the moment in rehab, after an attack, when a fellow patient proposed a metaphor describing how to deal with her disease. He told her: imagine you are tied to a big black dog that you must take care of for the rest of your life. You cannot cut it loose; you are attached to it until your very last day. But you have a choice: either you treat the dog well, and it might be friendly to you, or you neglect or mistreat it, and it will turn against you.

Hearing about this metaphor felt like an experience of discovery that had impressed the young woman. In a way it helped her from time to time. But it also still fascinated her, and she suspected it could be fruitful to explore the experience further to be open to its full potential. The Wonder Lab would structure this exploration by opening five 'spaces' (phenomenological space, hermeneutic space, a space for meeting with the experience of art and philosophy, existential space, space of phronesis), to disclose the full potential of the way the metaphor had touched her.

As forms of spiritual care, Wonder Labs integrate or presuppose all the elements we discussed before: inner space, resonance, unavailability, transformation, dealing with the weight of words, and suspending or bracketing our 'natural' understanding of the world. By doing so, they also connect with the poetical dimension of life celebrated in great works of art. Although philosophical by nature, Wonder Labs are far from merely intellectual or cognitive. They ask participants to be fully present to the phenomenon that is explored, with all their faculties and capacities.

Wonder Labs seem to be great places for opening and practicing a specific way of being in the world that fosters the humanization of health care. But they also take time and are possible only if people are willing to participate in a process that has an open and uncertain outcome. Not every health care professional is willing to engage in a transforming experience. In many instances, therefore, we might be happy when some of the Socratic virtues that Finn Hansen connects with Wonder Labs are present. Interestingly, they all have a connection with inner space, if we rephrase them in the following way: 1) *love* is making space for what is the dearest and most precious in your life; 2) *silence* is making space in order to hear what the heart, situation/relation calls you to say or think; 3) *humility* is making space to acknowledge the insufficiency of your own words and thoughts compared to the saturated meaningfulness you feel you are in resonance with; 4) *humor* is making space for new and unexpected perspectives that gently question the importance of your own perspective; 5) *courage* is making space for leaving your comfort zone and instinct for self-preservation; 6) *self-discipline* is making space to follow a tradition that can foster your growth in humaneness; 7) *friendship* is making space for being connected to a soul companion that follows you to your own limitations of thought and beyond, in search of the better person you aspire to become.

CONCLUSION

In this contribution, I have explored the humanization of health care with the metaphor of inner space as my starting point. After calling for a non-instrumental approach to spiritual care to connect to the human beings we are related to in caring practices, I analyzed Hartmut Rosa's concept of resonance in order to articulate the non-availability of the transformative process of humanizing health care. Having meditated on the weight of words, I argued that phenomenology can help us to go beyond words and reconnect to the underlying phenomena. Wonder Labs seem to be a balanced way of supporting this quest, simultaneously respecting the unavailability ('*Unverfügbarkeit*') of the process and structuring it in a way that is acceptable to a health care system obsessed with making the world 'visible, accessible, controllable, and usable' (Rosa, 2019, pp. 21–24).

REFERENCES

Carel, H. (2012). Phenomenology as a resource for patients. In: *The Journal of Medicine and Philosophy: A Forum for Bioethics and Philosophy of Medicine.* Vol. 37(2): pp. 96–113.

Carel, H. (2014). *Illness. The cry of the flesh* (revised edition). New York: Routledge.

Cobb, M., Puchalski, C.M. & Rumbold, B (eds.) (2012). *Oxford Textbook of Spirituality in Healthcare*. Oxford: University Press.

Hansen, F.T. (2015). The call and practice of wonder: how to evoke a Socratic community of wonder in professional settings. In: Weiss, N.M. (ed.), *Socratic handbook: Dialogue methods for philosophical practice* (pp. 217–44). Vienna: LIT Verlag.

Hansen, F.T. (2020). Learning to innovate in higher education through deep wonder. *Philosophy and Theory in Higher Education*. Vol. 1(3): pp. 51–74.

Leget, C. (2007). Retrieving the Ars moriendi tradition. *Medicine Health, Care and Philosophy.* Vol. 10(3): pp. 313–19.

Leget, C. (2016). A new art of dying as a cultural challenge. *Studies in Christian Ethics*. Vol. 29(3): pp. 279–85.

Leget C. (2017). *Art of Living, Art of Dying. Spiritual Care for a Good Death.* London and Philadelphia: Jessica Kingsley Publishers.

Leget, C. (2020). Forgiveness and reconciliation in palliative care: the gap between the psychological and moral approaches. *Religions*. Vol.11(9): pp. 440. doi:10.3390/rel11090440.

Mercier, P. (2020). *Das Gewicht der Worte*. München: Carl Hanser Verlag.

Puchalski C. et al. (2014). Improving the spiritual dimension of whole person care: Reaching national and international consensus. *Journal of Palliative Medicine*. Vol 17(6): pp. 642–56.

Rosa, H. (2016). *Resonanz. Eine Soziologie der Weltbeziehung*. Berlin: Suhrkamp.
Rosa, H. (2019). *Unverfügbarkeit*. Vienna: Residenz Verlag.
Sulmasy, D.P. (2006). *The rebirth of the clinic: an introduction to spirituality in health care*. Washington, D.C: Georgetown University Press.
Tronto, J.C. (1993) *Moral boundaries. A political argument for an ethic of care*. New York/London: Routledge.

Chapter 3

The Case and Its Moral Requirements

Solveig Botnen Eide

You (child welfare services worker) sit on my whole life story and you
have the power to make quite serious choices in my life,
so I at least deserve to feel that you care
and that you love me.

—(Ayla in Alexander proff, Gloria proff, Toresen, G. and I. Stenrem 2018, p. 12)

Leading thinking on moral obligation of professionals has so far been characterized by an understanding that it is the individual receiving help who requires moral attention, with particular focus on the person's vulnerability (Banks, 2006). I want to stop and wonder about what it means when Ayla indicates that the case itself, her life story, presents demands for care and love to the professionals.

She says that the child welfare worker sits on her whole life story, and that this fact represents demands on these professional. Her statement indicates that there is a connection between what the professionals are occupied with, their case, and ethical demand. As a phenomenon, her life story is understood and becomes visible for the child welfare professional. How can it be understood that a phenomenon involves and raises ethical demands?

The case itself and its demand is the focal point in this text. The overall aim of professional practice in health, education, and welfare is the best of the other. Even though those fields show great variation when it comes to concretization of this aim, they are all intertwined with people's own life, with their life stories. Inspired by Ludwig Wittgenstein (1998), I would state that the cases have character of life questions involved and inextricably linked in daily life, by Ayla illustrated by her life story, associated with care and love.

Although life questions basically can be said to entail something common to human beings, when we seek to understand them more closely, they will always be intertwined with a context. In this text, the context is child welfare as a public service. The discussions will primarily be related to this field and limited to what is often referred to as the "narrow" child welfare, i.e., the public activities that intervene when children are exposed to neglect, violence, and abuse (Berrick, 2018). Such interventions are deeply serious and require professional skills, knowledge, and legal legitimacy. Later in the text I will show that professional skills and psychological and legal knowledge have been given significant and increasing weight in the development of child welfare. Ayla's statements may, however, indicate that there are some features of the case itself that the professional and legal approaches do not capture.

My point of departure is in children and young people's own reflections of their experiences with child protection, starting with Ayla's quote. My main source for this is the book *Child Welfare from Us Who Know It*, in which children and young people write about their experiences with child welfare, documenting vital aspects of child welfare themes and showing how they are inextricably embedded in their life and linked to their life-world. They ask for trust, openness, love, and humanity (Forandringsfabrikken, 2019). My overall interpretation of their contributions is that they call for re-humanization or just humanization of child protection. Inspired with Harmut Rosa I will say that they point to a dissonance between the case and the child welfare service's handling of this (Rosa, 2020).

My aim is to shed light on the character of life issues as phenomenon emerging in professional work. How can we understand that the phenomenon itself has inherent moral demands, and what are such demands about? An elaboration of these points will constitute the main section of the chapter, but first I will give an introduction of the field of child welfare, with special emphasis on the need of re-humanization.

Humanization is in short about what it is being a human and an understanding that people have something in common, some core needs and core values. Those needs and values are a basis in professional work with people (Banks, 2006), but they may come under pressure and also be displaced by different techniques and approaches. Re-humanization is about a revitalization to this basis.

CHILD WELFARE SERVICE—IN NEED OF HUMANIZATION?

Is a re-humanization of child welfare service really needed? We will see that the service originated as a response to children's needs and vulnerabilities. The overriding goal is to take care of children. In this sense, both starting point and purpose are humanistic not only in their current form, but throughout the history of child welfare, as we will explore.

Care for children who are mistreated and/or not taken care of by their own parents or are orphaned, has ancient roots. Historically, relatives, other individuals, and religious and charitable organizations have responded to the distress of children and brought them to fostering situations (Schene, 1998). What is required in these situations to take care of children has changed. Modern child welfare stems from a centuries-old history. With modern child welfare I refer to child protection as a public matter (Berrick, 2018) and with the Norwegian child welfare as the key example I use. The foundation for intervention has been a moral obligation to take care of, and protect, neglected and/or abused children. Although it has been assumed that those who were to make decisions in such cases and those who take care of the children needed solid knowledge, it was also recognized that there were strong reasons based on everyday life knowledge and moral perceptions (Achtander and Dahstrøm, 1934, Eide 2007).

The response of society to this challenge of children vulnerable to neglect and abuse is visible in legislation and the creation of laws. The Norwegian Act on the Treatment of Neglected Children entered into force on January 1, 1900. It was drafted by Attorney General Bernhard Getz and was the first child welfare act, not only nationally, but also internationally. The target group was children vulnerable to neglect and abuse of various kinds. Shifts in thinking can be identified already in the first half of the last century. The field of welfare was gradually professionalized (Slagstad and Messel, 2014). Additionally, new fields of knowledge emerged, such as psychology and pedagogy. Gradually, more emphasis was placed on formal education providing special understanding of children. Within child welfare, challenges were increasingly met with psychological approaches.

Everyday knowledge and moral perceptions principles gradually lost influence in favor of these new forms of knowledge. I want to say that there were good reasons for this. The emergence of pedagogy and psychology cast critical light on brutal forms of child rearing, to name just one example. At the end of the last century, we also saw an increased emphasis on legal rights and legal protection, which must be understood in connection with the serious measures that child protection can implement, such as moving a child to a foster home against the will of those involved. Both psychological knowledge and legal protection have deep connections with caring for people, and so they represent humanizing features. This is particularly visible in the emergence of these dimensions in the history of child protection. The emergence of psychological knowledge can be seen as a reaction to brutal forms of upbringing. The increasing legalization can be seen against the background of intrusive measures in the lives of individuals without a sufficient legal basis. But could it also be that something has been lost? Can the understanding of children and their life stories become one-sidedly informed by psychological thinking and legal thinking without losing significant aspects? In the past decade we have seen reactions from those who have received help from child welfare services that may indicate that key human dimensions have been displaced.

THE CHILD WELFARE FIELD AND ITS CASE CONDITIONS

Child welfare is governed by legislation in which intervention criteria are specified. There are relatively large variations in child welfare legislation across countries, and not all countries have special laws regulating this field. In spite of the large variation in child welfare systems in different countries, it is nevertheless the case that the main target group is children who suffer injuries in their own homes. How their life is, the quality of the relationship with the parent, and day-to-day care are examples of conditions to be evaluated by child protection services. There is a complexity and seriousness in these questions, and everyday themes and at the same time, deep encroachments on people's privacy with possible major consequences for those involved. The different issues that child protection considers and the resulting efforts that are mobilized are tied to children's everyday lives and cannot be separated from it.

The child welfare's cases, which are inseparably tied to children's everyday life, are handled by child welfare workers, i.e., social workers with special competence linked to children and youth. The cases and questions presented by the children are handled by the child welfare workers. These cases have professional, administrative, and legal dimensions. When Ayla refers to "you," she means the workers who have been assigned to her case and have the responsibility to follow it up. As we have seen, Ayla gathers this under the concept of life story. She also mentions care and love, pervasive concepts in child protection, which she claims is something she can demand due to the fact that the child welfare sits on her whole life story. This appears to be a moral demand. Before we go into a more detailed look at what this demand entails, and how it can be understood, it is necessary to examine such phenomena, using care as a central example. Care is part of child welfare service's case conditions. It is an assessment theme when a child's care in the home is to be evaluated. It is a measure when the care is taken from the parents and given to the foster parents.

In Norwegian, as in other Germanic languages, we seek to address the phenomenon of care with concepts and words that are composed of care, concern, and grief (Caprona, 2013, p. 817). Concern and grief direct attention to the complexities of phenomena behind the English-language term "care." Child welfare service assess whether a child's care is good enough. They can take measures to improve care, for example, finding a foster home for the child. In the foster home, it is the foster parents who will provide for the child and care for it. Foster parents are in the parents' place. What is the nature of such care and its origin? Or, asked in a different way, where do we have to search to find the origin of care? A concept derives its content from outside itself, from a phenomenon to which it must apply in order to obtain relevant content (Blumer, 1954). This phenomenon that the concept seeks to cover and to which it must constantly return in order to be relevant, is what I call the concept's origin. Where do we need to focus our attention in order to give child welfare service's concept of care relevant content?

Care in child welfare is linked to children who are not well, to their vulnerability. It is about noticing, paying attention, and responding to other's vulnerabilities. Consequently, there is a connection between vulnerability and care. We often talk about "vulnerable groups," such as children in the child welfare system. This is how we can try to distance ourselves from our own vulnerability and under-communicate that it is a part of life, a part of our being in the world. It can also entail distancing from one's own vulnerabilities which can serve as a source of insight. Vulnerability is most deeply about the uniqueness of life (Løgstrup, 1997). This general vulnerability is about mortality, vulnerable phases of life with a particular focus on childhood, and it is about life lived in relationships, including unpredictable relationships (Løgstrup, 1997).

In the context of this chapter, it is the vulnerability of children and the relational side of life's vulnerability that is actualized. The child's vulnerability is often tied to age. The child has lived for a short time and consequently has limited skills and experience, which makes it vulnerable. Newborns are at the mercy of their environment. If this vulnerability is not responded to with care, the outcome is fatal. In the movement toward adulthood, the age-related vulnerability is gradually reduced. Vulnerability tied to relationships is also influenced by age, but not to the extent that we ever grow out of it.

We often talk about going in and out of different relationships. When Løgstrups writes about relationships as basic conditions, it means that, in the deepest sense, they are unavoidable (Løgstrup, 1971). A life in pure isolation is impossible. However, there are no guarantees associated with the various relationships in which a person is interwoven. Relationships can carry or break, or perhaps more realistically; they both carry and break, and break and carry. Care can be made more concrete in response to such risk factors. It is a response to something that is unmanageable for ourselves, and it manifests itself in different ways in different situations and relationships, and in different stages of life.

Since care is linked to vulnerability as a human condition, this gives it the character of being a foundation in our lives. Thus, care becomes fundamental and can be described as an existential condition (Heidegger, 2007, p. 201 et seq.; Vetlesen, 2001, p. 27 et seq.). We cannot live without care and although it is particularly visible in the early and late phases of life, it is profoundly phase-independent. As a response to the vulnerability we cannot avoid, caring is life-supportive and life-giving throughout the life course. In this way, it is dynamic and linked to our living conditions and our being in the world with others. We have addressed life itself, the vulnerability and entanglement as the origin of care, and the places we must seek to give care content.

Where does child welfare find content for the concept of care? We shall now return to child welfare services and a more detailed look at the concept of care. Where should one look to get a deeper understanding of what this term is all about? In child welfare, care has often been linked to practical tasks and to addressing specified psychological needs (Andersen, 2014; Vallesverd, 2018; Madsen, 2021). That is, one has primarily considered specific needs that are expected to be met in a child's home. This focus, and what is understood as good care, has primarily been linked to what one might call prevailing understandings and studies indicating that there is a correlation between the standard of good care, and the background of the professional. Middle class ideals are likely to set such standards (Kojan, 2011).

In recent decades those who have received care from child welfare service have raised their voices and received attention. Ayla is one of these voices. As I see it, her statemen is a source of a life-based understanding of what the term "care" refers to as we see it in the afore-referenced book from the Forandringsfabrikken (2019), Change Factory in English. From lived experiences the most important thing is that child welfare workers show love and care when working with children. This means that they are showing love by being kind in the way they are, speaking kindly, and showing emotion. With references to lived experience, they told us that they know they are talking to a person and not a robot when love and care are recognized (Forandringsfabrikken, 2019, p. 17). Here, the child welfare concept of care is informed by the experiences and reflections of those who have experienced it. Words like *love*, *openness*, and *trust* are central. The term *home* is the experience of living life with others. However, this home base of care is not the only source to today's child welfare system's understanding of care, and perhaps not the one of greatest influence.

Life-based understanding is an open position, open to different theoretical resources, including humanistic disciplines. The influence of psychology in the field has been increasing over the past decade (Madsen, 2021). Of course, there is not necessarily a contradiction between searching in a life experience perspective and searching in psychology as a subject field. It is nevertheless the case that psychology's treatment orientation emphasizes a clearer rationale and has a different form of goal management than is the case in experiences of living life at home, a statement to be elaborated on later in this text.

THE PHENOMENON ITSELF AND ITS INHERENT MORAL DEMAND

Let us return to Ayla's wording in the introductory quote. Here she says that she at least deserves care and love because child welfare services sits on her entire life story. We can imagine the following alternative formulation: since I am so vulnerable, I at least deserve care and love. The content of these formulations are close to each other, but present a different focus. While the alternative formulation draws attention to the person, Ayla's formulation draws attention to the subject matter, the phenomenon itself, which is in the hands of the child welfare workers. The phenomenon itself calls for moral attention. In the alternative formulation, it is Ayla as a vulnerable person who calls for moral attention.

To say that the phenomenon itself calls for moral attention, is to say that it is not neutral in a moral sense. To unpack this, what it means that the phenomenon itself has an inherent moral demand, we will turn to Løgstrup's work when he positions himself in contemporary thinking. In short, he argued that modern thinking entails a situation in which humans are imprisoned in their own heads. By this he means that a one-sided emphasis on the world and its phenomena as constructed (by humans) makes the world and the phenomena that surround us bereft of real values. As a consequence, shape and color, goals and meaning, good and evil, are phenomena that exist in our heads, and we give the world such qualities. In and of itself, the world and its phenomena are without goals and meaning. Consequently, the world and its phenomena have nothing to tell, nor does it present demands to us. This is where Løgstrup voices a different opinion (Christoffersen, 1999). In further development of his position within a phenomenological framework, he maintained that the world is real and that human beings are woven into a world that carries us with its ethical and aesthetic qualities (Løgstrup, 1971). This world is not constructed, but created and given to us, not once and for all, but in a lasting process in an endless struggle between life and death, between good and evil, hope and despair. The interpersonal features of life and our interactions with each other are inextricably linked to this struggle. Human life is in a complex way woven into reality and into relationships with other people, maintained as a basic condition, i.e., a condition we cannot change (Løgstrup, 1971, p. 20).

This means that the world and its phenomena are not neutral, nor do they simply represent a framework to be filled with value-based content. They have quite valuable content as a carrier with ethical and aesthetic content. This is a position challenged by the traditional distinction between is and ought, as we know it from David Hume's thinking. All normative content, our evaluations and the distinctions between right and wrong and evil and good, stem most deeply from ourselves and our position (Hume, 1969). In this sense, normativity has its origin in our interior selves, and not in the exterior world around us, in which we are interwoven. It means that we invent and construct values, they are not revealed, as we express it in Aristotelian thinking. Among newer thinkers who challenge the powerful tradition of Hume, we also find Hans Jonas. He is perhaps best known for his critique of anthropocentric ethics and the projection of nature as ethically relevant (Jonas, 1999). His thinking implies that what is valuable and worthy of protection, appears from something beyond and independent of cognitive activity. He uses newborn babies as an example. With its presence and its breath, a newborn directs itself towards the outside world—with its wordless imperative to be taken care of. Unless someone answers this challenge, the outcome is fatal, or to express it in Joan's words, the child's being is replaced by the non-being. From this Jonas deduces that our moral responsibility does not arise as a result of human intentionality, but rather as a result of the threatened position something or someone is in (Jonas, 1999). When Arendt writes about a related topic, she says that reality itself directs it's demands on us. She uses other words and writes, "claim on our thinking attention which all events and facts arouse by virtue of their existence" (Arendt, 2003, p. 160). The context from which this quotation is taken is a closer discussion of the impact that learned approaches and prevailing procedures have on our attention. Approaches and prevailing procedures have a directional influence on our attention. Approaches and prevailing procedures control our moral gaze so that morality is perceived as action and behavior in line with them. This involves a risk that the demands that reality itself directs at our thoughts will fall into a blind spot. This can be extremely risky because it can blind us to what is really at stake. Here she uses Adolf Eichmann as an example. In carrying out his mission for a final solution to the Jewish question, he followed the rules that followed the mission to the letter, with the result that he became blind to the demands reality made on him, namely that it was about other people's lives (Arendt, 2003).

This line of thinking has common ground with Løgstrup's notion that the world and what surrounds us is neither worthless nor mute, but express a demand against us that is independent of our value position. When Løgstrup addresses this topic, he writes that the phenomenological analysis is neutral, but not the phenomena it examines (Løgstrup, 1961/1995, p. 195). In his further work he connects tone and expectation. In the tone of the phenomenon, there is a built-in expectation of following up on the tone and through this, the distinctive features of the phenomenon. There is a need of a corresponding tone or frequency in the response. In social work literature, we find related thoughts.

The social worker is asked to tune into the frequency of their cases (Shulmann, 2009). As I interpret it, this is an implicit request to take the tone of the person involved and their case. That a phenomenon has tone means, as explored above, that it is not a neutral quantity. "I" is the social worker who is to take the tone set by the case in front of them, in Ayla's case, the child welfare worker. This is how I understand it, a thought that is inextricably linked to what Løgstrup points out, that life expresses itself. The phenomenon, in our case Ayla's life story and care, is not passively and unilaterally open to our interpretation, but directs demands towards us. It is not primarily a requirement to engage the phenomenon for further assessment, but to be touched or affected by it so that the response corresponds with the phenomenon's uniqueness and tone. What tone or mood can we say that Ayla's life story has? We do not know much about it other than that it is in the hands of child welfare services. This indicates moments of vulnerability that extend beyond the vulnerability one might otherwise find in a young person's life story. Ayla further says that it is the whole life story and its demands on child welfare services is that they at least love her. I think Ayla touches on something very central in her understanding of life history. It is an expression of lived life—in small and large portions—and it is an expression of a person, who evokes a response that exists in the interpersonal repertoire as we formulate it when someone is to meet us all and have a significant influence on our future; then at least there must be someone who wishes us well and loves us. In order to come to a more intimate understanding of the fact that the phenomenon itself has inherent moral requirements, it may be appropriate to look at the relationship between case and person. I will continue to use Ayla as an example.

Let's again turn back to the introduction and Alya's statement and my alternative wording. I point out that these two statements have different focus but are still related to each other. They both deal with Ayla. She points to her story and the alternative formulation points to Ayla, the main person in the story. If we connect to care, we can say that the first formulation connects to care, while the second connects to the girl who needs care. This shows how the field of child welfare services is inextricably linked to the life of others, and to lived life. It relates to broad concepts that cannot be determined in content in the form of delimiting definitions. This is how they have the character of being life-value phenomena, and this is how, as we shall see in the next section, they claim to have a built-in dynamic that is more than causality.

LIFE STORY, LOVE, AND CARE

Becoming acquainted with Ayla and her life story presents a demand, as Ayla sees it, a demand to the child welfare workers for care and love. "We cannot say what life is like, just tell the story," writes Arendt (1971/Heberlein, 2021, p. 190). The life story, which can consist of many or few fragments, is about our experiences as we remember them. Which memories are central may change over time. Some memories will be able to have a more prominent position than others and set both theme and tone that lasts, other memories will have a more transient character, but can still emerge in consciousness again and again, in new ways. When we tell these stories and when they are told, we are, as it were, evoking our own identity, that is, ourselves. The main point here is not that our identity, the core of our self, is constructed by our storytelling, but that our identity is evoked and interpreted by telling our life story.

The stories about experiences can be adjusted and changed as our understanding of ourselves are changing. The main character of a life story will be the individual the story is about. It will (of course) also include other people and the context in which the story takes place, but still with the main character is the vantage point and center for interpreting the participation of others and the significance of the context. In child welfare and as Ayla refers to the phenomenon of life history, it is terms of intervention in her everyday life. And the child welfare service "sits on" not only her story, but also on her.

Is the reformulation of Ayla's statement superfluous? Perhaps it was superfluous in the sense that the reflections on the two statements (see page 7) showed that directing moral focus on life history and on the person is, by and large, the same thing. The gaze that is directed towards life history is directed towards the person. Anyone who is moved by a life story is moved by a person. It is nevertheless the case that by reformulating and going closer to the core of the formulations, we reveal that cases in the child welfare service are morally demanding. Cases are inextricably linked to the lives of children and young people and, woven into their everyday lives and existence—their life histories. What can we say about the demands for response that are built into the child welfare service's case, in the life histories of children and young people? The response must correspond with the nature of the case as a world-life phenomenon. We have seen that care is a part of the world of life, inextricably linked to our lives. Heidegger illuminates this when he says that care is an existential condition (Heidegger, 2001). Care is, as we have seen, a key concept in child welfare professional literature and in the legislation that regulates child protection activities. But what about love? Unless love is new in child welfare, the concept of love seems to be revitalized. We find love both implicitly and explicitly in the history of child welfare: Implicit in the requirement that foster parents accept the foster child as their own. Explicit in "upbringing with love" a term taken from the *Journal of Parents and Children* from 1902 and which child psychologist Olav Tiller highlights in his account of the history of childhood. In the magazine Tiller refers to, the importance of upbringing love is demonstrated. Love is seen as tool for upbringing of children as good people. He emphasized this love as particularly important for children who have experienced neglect, i.e., child welfare system children, since their upbringing has been deficient (Tiller, 2000, p. 78). This concept is in content close to what we find in the English debate about love in child welfare system around "tough love" when arguing for a strict upbringing, but still love (Bradt and Bouverne-De Bie, 2009). Rather than holding an innate value, love seems to be a tool in child rearing. Loving practices become disciplinary practices (Tharan, 2018). Here the meaning of love seems to extend beyond itself and become a tool.

I will return to that issue, but first, let us examine the phenomenon of love more closely. I start by asking questions, as we did in the case of care. How can we search for the phenomenon the concept is meant to cover and provide information on? What experiences can contribute to creating content for the concept? Reservations about using the concept in child welfare have been that it is a concept from an intimate private sphere—often connected to sexuality. This form of love—eros—is a form of love which connects two humans in a special way, where both to the same degree are dependent on each other, the interests of one coincide with those of the other. Arendt talks of love—eros—in a similar fashion. In Vita Activa (1958), she writes that between these two who love each other there is no "in-between." When she reflects on what it entails to lose your husband and life partner, she writes that the world they created and where they felt at home was destroyed and no longer existed after Heinrich died (Herberline, 2021). From this perspective, we can state that the concept of love seeks its meaning in the strongest experiences of belonging. But what about love in relations to other persons, the love we describe as neighborly love? What experiences can shed light on this concept? When Jesus speaks of this phenomenon (in the Bible), he says that we should love our neighbor, our fellow human beings, as we love ourselves. Thus, love of oneself and personal experience are introduced to grasp the meaning of neighborly love. To Arendt, it seems like an important point that the very connection to oneself and our own wellbeing cannot be separated from our own interests—and cannot be without selfishness. Løgstrup does not regard this point of loving our self as an objection. He is arguing that connecting with loving our self and own experiences rather than making neighborly love self-centered radicalizes it.

The other, my neighbor, has the same need for love that I myself have. Consequently, the concept of love, similarly to care, go to life experiences to create content, toward what I (inspired by Løgstrup) will call life-opening phenomena, creating a contrast to clearly definable phenomena with clear borders.

WHAT KIND OF ACTION IS CALLED FOR?

We have seen that care is a key issue in child protection. This is observable in policy as well as professional literature for child protection workers. Even though the child protection care concept has been tied to love, the concept of love has until quite recently been peripheral. Nevertheless, it is interesting that the concept of love now is embedded in Norwegian child welfare law, as a direct result of the child protection children's efforts. The law states that the children should be met by safety, love, and understanding. The requirement is not limited to persons serving as substitute parents as foster parents, but is also tied to everybody who, through child protection service meets children and youth. This means that the concept is on its way into professional practice and sets a standard for work to be done. So far, in several parts of this text, I have mentioned that the phenomena of care and love sets a tone and inherent demands; they require what I call action. In this last chapter, we examine what type of action is called for.

How a term is filled with content and meaning is dependent on where we look for the content, which phenomena one is looking for. Child Protection is, as I have mentioned, strongly influenced by the field of psychology. Different psychological treatment orientations tend to emphasize ideals that they have in common with care, such as life-world phenomena, trust, openness, and respect. These are phenomena that are all related to love. There is therefore reason to ask whether the gap between professional work and the life phenomena involved can become bridged. To get closer to an answer to this question, I want to look more closely at the rationales of care and treatment. Treatment can go a long way in translating such life-world phenomena into therapeutic tools. We shall see that there is a rewrite which also involves a reduction. Knud E. Løgstrup writes extensively about the risks involved in making phenomena that are related to relationships and trust into means

(Løgstrup, 1972). Inspired by Løgstrup I would argue that the same is the case with care and love and as a phenomenon, they cannot be turned into a pure means without losing peculiar character. When I write pure means, it is to show that (of course) it can also be the case that we provide care for a more concrete purpose, such as helping children control their anger. But care is, as we have seen, more extensive than this. We can point to elements that are part of it, elements that are often age- and context-dependent, but we cannot give it a definitive definition without the risk of reducing it. Care and associated phenomena are at risk of being perverted if they are subjected to an instrumental and objectifying attitude. We can use trust as an example. If trust becomes a pure means, for example when a child welfare worker uses it to get a youth to change his mind in line with the child welfare view, there will be a slippery transition from trust to manipulation. In this way, trust can lose its character as trust and ultimately be perverted.

It means that the phenomena call for a response beyond the purely instrumental.

A pure instrumental response arises out of an instrumental logic in which one does something with the other in order to achieve a certain result. There is a logic of action that corresponds to what Hannah Arendt calls production, which she contrasts with action (1958, p. 192 ff). What separates the action from the production? In production, use is made of suitable tools. These can be material, as in the carpenter's toolbox. They can also be intangible and in the form of good questions in the psychologist's toolbox. Tools are used for a specific purpose to achieve a specific result. This means that the use of tools is associated with a causally oriented rationale where one thinks that a particular action or intervention has a predictable result. The result of the production has a set path beforehand. If you just follow a recipe or procedure, results are achievable. When this logic unilaterally applies to other people, it suggests a form of human labor that is supposed to bring about changes in people, with results envisioned before work began. One does something with the other in the sense that the activity is one-way.

It is nevertheless true that one with a humanistic perspective as a starting point, can never disregard that such work is never one-way and therefore not fully predictable. It is always interwoven in relations with another human being, in our relationship to the child who also exerts their influence. We can hope that caring actions have good consequences, but effects of actions in an Arendsk sense are not predictable as is the effect of production. They avoid statistical calculation. Also, the one who gives the child care is challenged, pressed, recognized and confirmed in the act of care. This leads to the question of why we should show care and provide care, and why we should love one another. The answer is that we concern one another. This is how care has a moral justification. Both action and attitude are included in the concept. The rooting of care and love in our life world and in the moral domain lends itself to linguistic expressions, expressions that embrace closeness, intersubjectivity, and responsibility. The language of care expresses a moral awareness of being involved in the lives of others and taking care of their well-being.

These phenomena will demand different actions, depending on what is at risk, but it is the actions and approaches required have one thing in common: to be open and touched by the other's situation—an open gaze for each individual child—for everything living that has a face.

REFERENCES

Andersen, I. L. (2014). Traumebevisst tilnærming. In S. Søftestad & I. L. Andersen (red.) Seksuelle overgrep mot barn. Traumebevisst tilnærming (s. 54–62). Oslo: Universitetsforlaget.

Arendt, H., J. V Scott, and J. C. Stark (1996). Love and Saint Augustine. University of Chicago Press.

Arendt, H. (1959). The human condition. New York: A Doubleday Anchor Book. New York.

Arendt, H. (2003). Some Questions of Moral Considerations. In J. Kohn (red) Responsibility and judgement. New York: Schocken Books.

Arctander, S. og S: Dahlstrøm (1934). Hvordan går det våre vergerådsbarn? En statistisk studie bygget på erfaringer fra Oslo Vergeråd 1900–1928. Oslo: Olaf Norlis Forlag.

Banks, S: (2006). Ethics and value in social work. London: Palgrave Macmillan. Basingstoke.

Berrick, J. D. (2018). The impossible imperative navigating the competing principles of child protection. Oxford: Oxford University Press.

Blumer, H. (1954). What is wrong with social theory? *American Sociological Review,* 18, 3–10.

Bradt, L. and Bouverne-De Bie (2009). Social Work in a Shift from Welfare to Justice. *British Journal of Social Work*, 3, pp. 113–27.

Christoffersen, S. Aa. (1999). Etikk, eksistens og modernitet. Innføring i Løgstrups tenkning. Oslo: Tano Ashenpoug.

Caprona, Y. D. (2013). Norsk etymologisk ordbok. Oslo: Kagge forlag.

Eide, S. B. (2007). Prinsipper og levd liv. Doktorgradsavhandling. Universitetet i Oslo.

Forandringsfabrikken (2019). Barnevernet fra oss som kjenner det. Oslo: Forandringsfabrikken kunnskapssenter.

Heberlein, A. (2021). hannah arendt. Oslo: Cappelen Damm.

Heidegger, M. (2007). Væren og tid. Oslo: Pax Forlag.

Hume, D. (1969). An Inquiry into Human Nature. Harmondsworth: Penguin, 1969.

Jonas, H. (1999). Teknikk, medisin og etikk. Oslo: Cappelen upopulære serie.

Kojan, B. H. (2011). Klasseblikk på et barnevern i vekst. Doktorgradsavhandling, NTNU.

Løgstrup, K. E. (1956/1997). The ethical demand. University of Notre Dame Press. Notre Dame and London.
Løgstrup, K. E. (1961). Etik og kunst. København: Gyldendal.
Løgstrup, K. E. (1997). System og Symbol. Gyldendal, København.
Løgstrup, K. E. (1971). Etiske begreber og problemer. Gyldendal, København.
Madsen, O. J. (2017). Den terapeutiske kulturen. Oslo: Universitetsforlaget.
Rosa, H. (2020). Resonance. A Sociology of our relationship to the world. Cambridge: Polity Press, Oslo.
Schene, P. A. (1998). Past, Present and Future Roles of Child Protective Service. *The Future of Children*, April 1, 1998, Vol. 8 (1), pp. 23–38.
Slagstad, R. and T. Messel. (2014). Profesjonshistorie. Oslo, Pax forlag.
Thrana, H.M. (2018). Kjærlighet. I Ask, T. og S. B. Eide. (red.). Barnevernets begreper i bevegelse. Oslo: Gyldendal akademisk.
Tiller, P. O. (2000). Studier i barndom. Kristiansand: Høyskoleforlaget.
Vallesverd, V. U. (2018). Omsorgssvikt. I T. Ask og S. B. Eide (red.).Barnevernets begreper i bevegelse. Oslo: Gyldendal.
Vetlesen, A. J. (2001). Omsorg-mellom avhengighet og autonomi. I K. W. Ruter & A. J.
Vetlesen (red.). Omsorgens tvetydighet (s. 27–40). Oslo: Gyldendal Akademisk.
Wittgenstein, L. (1998). Ludwig Wittgeinstein. Den ukjente dagboken. Oversatt av Amåls, K. Oslo: O. Spartacus forlag.

Chapter 4

Perspectives on the Wonders of Sovereign Life Utterances and Care Ethics

Åshild Slettebø

In this chapter, I consider the phenomena of life utterances and the importance of understanding and respecting them in health care encounters. Life utterances are phenomena which describe natural ways of relating during encounters with other persons. It is how life utters itself. Løgstrup (2013) mentions examples of sovereign life utterances in the form of phenomena such as trust, openness of speech, compassion, and mercy. What characterizes life utterances and why are they important in nursing care? Vulnerability is an emotion experienced by many patients within the health care sector. It begins in the assessment/diagnostic phase and continues through treatment until rehabilitation and recovery, or until the condition becomes chronic or the patient succumbs to their illness. My question, then, is whether this vulnerability aligns with the "existential-phenomenological dialogical wondering theory" of this book or whether it violates it or raises some challenges? Hansen and Jørgensen (2020) examine Heidegger's concept of an "existential homecoming" focusing on resonance with being and not on interpersonal and psychological relations. They argue that a wonder-based approach is essential for establishing openness, trust, and attentiveness in nurse-patient relationships. While I agree with this approach, this chapter seeks to delve further into the understanding of resonance and relationships in nurse-patient encounters and argues that this approach can potentially improve the relationships in nursing care.

I rely on Danish theologian K. E. Løgstrups's (2013) understanding of life utterances and on the Norwegian nursing philosopher Kari Martinsen's

(1991; 2012) reflections on care ethics and insights into how these utterances are fundamental for nursing care for the vulnerable patient and for humanizing health care encounters. Furthermore, I explore nurse theorist Joyce Travelbee's Human-to-Human Relationship Model (1971) in which Travelbee argues that there should not be a patient-nurse relationship in health care services and nursing, but rather a human-to-human meeting. I will consider how such a relationship evolves in the context of Løgstrup's understanding of life utterances.[1]

My contribution lies within what is written in the introduction chapter: "Løgstrup's notion of the 'Spontaneous and Sovereign Life Utterances' (Løgstrup, 2013) can indeed be seen as ethical and ontological 'spheres of resonance' in the midst of daily life and as metaphysical experiences, which are 'on the outside of modernity.'" Thus, I want to add to nursing philosophy the notion of sovereign life utterances as important in establishing resonant relationships in nursing care. Furthermore, I want to address how respecting these life utterances may open up a space for what is 'unavailable' in the encounter of human beings, which is the key to the humanization of health care professions and the flourishing of humanity.

In this chapter, I explore the following questions: What is the difference between being in a *relation* and being in *resonance* with another person or the world? Can one be in a relation with a life phenomenon, or would it be more accurate to say that one can only be in resonance with it? Is it possible to be in resonance with a 'vulnerable' patient without having a relationship and being in a relation with that patient? I use the work of Hartmut Rosa (2019) and his book on resonance, *Resonance: A Sociology of Our Relationship to the World,* to address these questions.

A STORY FROM CLINICAL NURSING PRACTICE

I want to begin this exploration of life utterances and care ethics with an experience I had working as a nurse at a nursing home. During the night shift, I was in charge of the entire nursing home, which consisted of four floors with approximately thirty residents each. One evening at ten o'clock, when my shift began, the evening shift nurse and a physician from the acute center in the city briefed me on the status of one of the residents who had fallen earlier in the evening and was being treated. They checked her for a hip fracture but did not find any signs of one, so she was given a painkiller and put to bed. After a couple of hours, I was called to check on this patient because she was complaining of pain. She had a diagnosis of dementia, and it was difficult to understand what she said and meant, but we could tell that she was in severe pain. I also checked the hip and could not see any physical signs of fracture.

Still, I was concerned about her behavior and discomfort. I decided to contact the ambulance and send her to the hospital for an X-ray. When the paramedics arrived, they laughed at me and said, "There is no fracture, but we will take her to the hospital since you are so persistent." Later that morning, before I went off duty, they called from the hospital and said, "It's a good thing you sent her to X-ray as there is a hip fracture that needs to be operated on immediately."

PERSPECTIVES RELATED TO CARING SCIENCE

I have often wondered about this situation. After that night, I later wondered what it was that made me decide to send her to the hospital, despite everyone agreeing that there were no clear physical signs of fracture. I have since thought that it was something in her eyes and her gaze that cried for help and communicated wordlessly that the pain was unbearable, and something was really wrong. Her eyes were filled with a sort of anxiety, conveying to me that she was frightened by what she was experiencing, even though she could not understand or explain it. I also think my choice resulted from spending some time with her before deciding what to do. I did not just do the physical examination; I also tried talking with her to communicate at a level that could be understood by a person with dementia who had difficultly expressing herself. One example of her attempts to communicate was when she burst out with, "Who turned on the winter here?" I realized that she had the beginning stages of hypothermia, and that also alerted me that there was something wrong in her body that she was unable to directly express.

Nursing professor Kari Martinsen has written about how caring is fundamental in nursing (Martinsen, 1991). Caring as a phenomenon is threefold: it is relational, it is practical, and it is moral (Martinsen, 1991, pp. 14–17). Caring as a relational phenomenon always occurs between at least two partners, the caregiver, and the care receiver. As a practical phenomenon, caring is always about a task or something that the caregiver does for the care receiver. It could be as practical as helping with meals or bathing, and it could be sitting beside the care receiver to talk or provide comfort. This means caring as a relational phenomenon is about the caregiver having concern for the care receiver's needs. According to Martinsen (1991), the moral aspect of caring is the obligation for the caregiver to take responsibility for the vulnerable. In the caring relationship, the caregiver has autonomy and power, and the care receiver is the one in need. The Norwegian philosopher and professor Arne Johan Vetlesen (2001) says that the care receiver's position is one of unwanted dependency (p. 37). The person has not chosen to be ill or to require care. They may even experience a sense of being coerced into a situation of dependence and unwillingly restrained due to their illness. Often, the care receiver is in an unfamiliar institutional environment such as a hospital or nursing home. The nurses and other health care personnel have chosen their profession and are, in a sense, "at home" in a self-selected environment. This implies an asymmetric relationship between caregivers and care receivers. The nurse or health care professional should advocate for the care receiver's right to optimal care, especially when they are in a vulnerable position. It is important that the moral aspect of caring respects the care receiver's integrity and vulnerability (Slettebø & Fredriksson, 2015).

SPONTANEOUS LIFE UTTERANCES

In his book *Settlement with Kierkegaard* (2013), Danish theologian and philosopher K.E. Løgstrup reflects upon the concept of "spontaneous life utterances." According to Løgstrup, these are phenomena that are so basic to our lives that we do not take note of them until they fail. Life utterances is a specific philosophical phenomenon that describes how we naturally meet each other in life encounters. Sovereign life utterances are characterized by mutuality and being intertwined with each other's lives. A hidden desire drives the tendency to fulfill an ethical demand that we all have towards other persons when we meet. The ethical demand is an unspoken request to be respected and taken care of in every encounter between two persons.

According to Løgstrup, there are some common signs for identifying life utterances such as openness of speech, trust, and mercy (2013). First, they are spontaneous, which means we do not determine whether we should meet a person from the life utterances they express in the situation. Second, they are sovereign; they appear by themselves in our daily dealings with one another. We do not create or control them, but they are instantaneously communicated by us. This implies that we trust one another spontaneously. It is not a premeditated decision, rather it is natural for us when meeting another person. Third, life utterances are silent and anonymous. They are not used as principles that can be verbal utterances; instead, their content is based on our perception and tangible experience of a situation. Fourth, life utterances are definitive, which means they are either in the situation or they are not. Fifth, and last, life utterances are radical, which means they are not indifferent to us. It matters whether I am faced with openness and trust or suspicion and mistrust. Each person must always consider whether we are willing to facilitate another person's life opportunities (Løgstrup, 2013). Løgstrup (2013) provides examples of sovereign life utterances in the form of phenomena such as trust, openness of speech, compassion, mercy, hope, and respect.

It can be problematic when a patient does not react towards the health care personnel with sovereign life utterances but with the opposite, which Løgstrup (2013, p. 95) calls circular life utterances. These include phenomena such as insults, jealousy, and/or envy. When primarily expressing circular life utterances, the focus is placed on one's own needs and feelings. The person's thoughts revolve around the perceived offenses they feel they have suffered or a lack of trust in the person with which they are interacting. Conversely, for spontaneous and sovereign life utterances, the focus is on the issue at hand, and both parts react spontaneously with trust and openness of speech. In this case, one is only suspicious and mistrusting if there are separate reasons not to be open and trusting; for example, they may react this way if they have experienced the other person lying about the issues at hand. This will harm the relationship, and it will not be a resonant or a human-to-human relationship.

Sovereign life utterances were present in the previously described situation about the female patient with the fractured hip, and their impact caused me to respond to her vulnerability. Although her presentation was wordless, a lot was communicated by her combined silence and the spontaneous presentation of her pain through her actions and expression. It was my perception of the situation that led to my decision to disobey the physician's order and to instead respond to the expression in the woman's eyes, just so she could receive medication for her obvious pain. She was not indifferent to me, and I felt she relied on me and trusted me. It was up to me to preserve this trust. In addition to being a responsible nurse and health care worker, I knew tacitly[2] that I had an ethical demand in that situation.

As Løgstrup writes in his book *The Ethical Demand* (1991, p. 24), an ethical demand is tacit and unspoken and consists of one individual embracing the other as they are by picking up on the other's voice and tone. In addition, the encounter between the vulnerable female patient and myself as the caregiver can be considered a resonant relationship. Rosa (2019) writes about both the voice and the eye/gaze and how they signal different forms of relationships:

> The human voice can also be said to express a person's *mood* (in German: *Stimmung*)—we may describe someone's voice as shaky, halting, gloomy, bright, ice cold (i.e., without resonance), husky (i.e., obscuring resonance), shrill, joyful, etc.—and this is all the more true of a person's *eyes*, their *look* or *gaze*, which likewise reveals their (momentary as well as fundamental) relationship to the world. . . . The most direct physical way to consciously establish a relationship with another human being, . . . is to make eye contact with it to *look it in the eye.* (Rosa, 2019, p. 66)

The female patient's gaze alerted me that her relationship with the world was distorted. It was not her usual expression, and I responded to the vulnerability that was present in her eyes. She looked me in the eye and silently expressed her pain and asked for help in what I will call a resonant way. By the "resonant way," I here experienced as a tacit way of relating to me as a nurse. This was by her non-verbal signs and gaze filled with anxiety. Her non-verbal cry for help indicated that she trusted me and the other health care personnel in the ward, and this trust can be considered a sovereign life utterance, as described by Løgstrup (2013).

It is important to consider the role that trust plays in the human-to-human relationship in nursing. Scholars have long debated whether trust is a prerequisite for a relationship or if it is the result of the nurse's hard work (Slettebø, 2012). The first form of trust is spontaneous trust, where one immediately meets the other with the confidence necessary to help them (Løgstrup, 2013). The second form of trust increases as it is earned. A phenomenological understanding, which Løgstrup defends, is that trust is a spontaneous life utterance in a relationship, and it has been suggested as a prerequisite for establishing relationships. Nurses must develop professional ethics where immediate trust is generated and responded to in a respectful manner. Thus, earned trust is cultivated and another aspect of trust needed for going forward.

Care should be ethically provided to receivers. This means that the caregiver respects the care receiver's vulnerability and earns their trust. Vetlesen (2010) says that to trust another is to leave someone—that is, the trusting person—to the caregiver. It is not to leave something in the hands of the other, as this "thing" can only be handled as an entity, rather than a human being. This may produce challenges because if trust is abused, the moral aspect of caring is not respected.

This argument is supported by the research of Jerak-Zuiderent (2015), which emphasizes that accountability in care relationships is "from somewhere and for someone" and not an accountability where care belongs to another domain in health care. This emphasis on the interweaving of accountability and caring shifts the focus from good care to meaningful care. Jerak-Zuiderent argues that there has been a divide between accountability and caring, where accountability has gone "from nowhere to everyone." This is not in line with a caring attitude in which the patient is a unique person to the caregiver (Jerak-Zuiderent, 2015). Therefore, she introduces the importance of seeing the care receiver as "someone," meaning to see them as a person in their own right. This may provide some insight into how I acted towards my patient. I saw her as someone in pain and I felt accountable to address her cry for help by providing her with the necessary care.

Caring means having concern for the other person, and it should create possibilities for the improved health and extended life of the care receiver. Tronto (2016) elaborates on the concept of care by identifying the following four dimensions: 1) caring about, which means to meet a patient's needs; 2) caring for, which means to accept responsibility and to realize when something must be done; 3) caregiving, which means a need has been identified and responsibility has been taken to meet that need; and 4) care receiving, which means the response of the care receiver to the care provided (p. 2). The caregiver must understand the care receiver's vulnerability and meet their needs in order to respect their trust. Care is experienced as a phenomenon that relieves a situation in which a patient is vulnerable. As I interpreted the situation presented at the beginning of this chapter, the female patient's trust would have been broken if I had failed to respond to the needs she was communicating. The patient's vulnerability led me to identify those needs and to act contrary to the physician's order since the patient's pain indicated to me that more care was needed than just providing painkillers.

Engster (2018) points out the importance of focusing on vulnerability in caring rather than on dependence. He argues that even if dependent individuals are included within the definition of care, care should be "framed more broadly to encompass all sorts of human vulnerability" (p. 8). Thus, dependence is an aspect of vulnerability, and other aspects of vulnerability must also be considered in addition to dependability. Kittay (2020) also considers vulnerability and the moral nature of dependency relations in caring relationships.

> It must be said that an individual has an unqualified obligation to assume the responsibilities of dependency work when the following conditions are met: 1) the needs are basic; 2) the vulnerability is extensive; and 3) the prior relation, which puts a particular individual into the position of having to assume such a vulnerability-responsive obligation has a moral warrant. Furthermore, this obligation has to be assumed even when there is a substantial cost to the dependency worker's own interests and projects. (Kittay, 2020, pp. 64–65)

Thus, Kittay (2020) argues that care requires some level of sacrifice from the caregiver. Van Nistelrooij and Leget (2017) discuss the costs and self-sacrifice involved in caring relationships and they challenge Carol Gilligan's (1982) theory of mature care in nursing. Gilligan theorizes that women conceptualize themselves as well as their morality. Women's morality causes them to care about and have concern for others as well as themselves, which impacts how they view themselves. According to Gilligan (1982), these elements of self and morality are interdependent in moral development. The care elements within Gilligan's theory are care for the other, care for oneself, and lastly balanced care for both the other and oneself in a caring encounter (1982).

However, Van Nistelrooij and Leget (2017) challenge Gilligan's assertion, by arguing that "moral questions involve sacrifice and guilt as inescapable in the choice's life forces upon people. . . . We, however, believe it central to the care-ethical epistemological claim that practices are the primary source of moral knowledge" (p. 701). Thus, they emphasize that the theoretical dichotomization of self-sacrifice and selfishness in mature care suggested by Gilligan (1982) must be problematized and related to empirical concepts of mature care.

As Kittay (2020) argues, a caring relationship involves self-sacrifice because a care receiver is not only dependent but also vulnerable. In my case, my decision did not involve much self-sacrifice, even though I risked being sanctioned by my superiors because I had opposed the physician's order and sent the patient for an X-ray. The patient was dependent on me, but it was her vulnerability that made me act despite the claims from all other care providers that she could not have broken her hip when she fell.

These reflections on caring relationships and moral development suggest the need for the humanization of care, as this book on "wonder and silence" advocates. By advocating for a humanistic shift in care, one transcends superficial caring experiences by creating a fundamental human-to-human relationship throughout the caring encounter.

HUMAN-TO-HUMAN RELATIONSHIP IN HEALTH CARE

I further wonder how Løgstrup's sovereign life utterances can promote more human-to-human relationships in health care. When describing the development of human-to-human relationships in nursing, nursing theorist, Joyce Travelbee (1971) explains that we experience several conflicts throughout our lives and that we are all accountable for the choices we make in our lives. Our responsibility includes loving each other as expressed through our actions towards those we encounter (Kierkegaard, 2013). Kierkegaard describes loving one another as an obligation to our neighbors. However, this obligation must not be understood within the context of duty ethics. It is a kind of moral obligation that serves as an ethos of care in the encounters between caregiver and care receiver.

When a patient tells their nurse that they are grateful for the help they received and the nurse answers that it was only their duty to help, this response may be equivalent to a friend visiting a patient at the hospital and emphasizing that they are only there out of duty and not because of their fondness for the patient. The patient may be somewhat hurt by such a response. However, if the nurse adds, "and it is my pleasure to do this for you as a wonderful and unique person whom I truly care for," the patient may feel better. This message establishes that caregiver and receiver are in a human-to-human relationship where they meet as two individuals with equal rights to respect, but with different levels of vulnerability and situational responsibilities. This can be then be considered a caring relationship where the two individuals are in resonance and experiencing sovereign life utterances in action. This is in line with Martinsen's (2012) statement that a nurse should have their heart in the caring relationship and not only rely on norms and duties (p. 104).

It often takes time to establish a relationship. Travelbee (1971) describes five phases in relationship development: Phase one is the meeting where a connection is immediately established between the two persons. Phase two is the emergence of personal identities, where both persons attempt to relate to one another as human beings and try to find meaning in their encounter. In this emergence, the two persons (e.g., the nurse and the patient) see each other as unique individuals independent of their situational roles. This is an important step according to Travelbee (1971) because situational roles hinder the possibility of meeting as individual humans with unique personalities, expectations, wishes, and needs. Phase three is empathy, where humans share in and relate to one another's experiences. Phase four is sympathy, which generates the desire to relieve or lessen another human's suffering (Travelbee, 2013). This is not a sentimental form of sympathy but rather an actionable sympathy that leads to meeting the other's needs and relieving their pain. Finally, stage five is rapport, which Travelbee defines as follows:

> A process, a happening, an experience between two persons. It may not be a mutual affair at first, but the sharing of the experience and participation in it grows as each individual unfolds him or herself in the interpersonal situation. . . . Rapport is a dynamic, fluctuating affair and it will change as changes occur in the interpersonal situation or relationship. (1963, p. 70)

Travelbee's concept of human-to-human relationships in nursing, in which the individuals have reached a level of "rapport," can be understood as a resonant relationship, as described by Rosa (2019). Based on these conceptual understandings, I argue that nursing can be humanized beyond its current use of standardized "packages" and terminology (e.g., The International Classification of Nursing Practice [ICNP]). In the case described above, I viewed the female patient as a unique individual with her own vulnerability and innate human rights. I had to address her pain in some way, and I knew that painkillers alone were not sufficient. I could not rely solely on the physical examination because it did not reveal what the problem was, and I risked losing the patient's trust since she was visibly experiencing severe pain that needed to be relieved. The standard package did not work in this instance and I had to establish a human-to-human resonant relationship with the female patient. Her trust led me to react by taking her pain seriously and doing more than was recommended by her physician.

According to Travelbee (1971), the phases in a human-to-human relationship are linear. This is because there can only be one first meeting and first impression upon which the relationship is built and through which emerging personal identities are established. However, later in the process, it may be possible to switch between empathy, which is being resonant, and sympathy, which is feeling what the other is experiencing and being motivated to act on their behalf. It is also possible to then return to understanding the experience as it develops. I believe that the development of human-to-human resonant relationships relies on life utterances in action. If the individuals in the situation do not have mutual trust, openness of speech, compassion, mercy, hope, and respect for one other, the attempt to develop an authentic relationship will fail, or the relationship will only exist within the nurse-patient paradigm. Therefore, I recommend adding a dimension to Travelbee's (1971) theory of human-to-human relationship that includes being resonant throughout relationship development and ongoing caring encounters.

RELATIONSHIP OR RESONANCE IN CARING?

I wonder whether being in a human-to-human relationship could be the same as being in resonance with each other, as presented in this book. I am puzzled by what the notion of being "in resonance" could mean other than being in a relationship. One may wonder about being in resonance with life phenomena rather than being in a relationship. Is it possible to be in resonance with a vulnerable person in health care without having established a human-to-human relationship with them? And is it possible to experience life phenomena within a caring situation without having relationships as axes of resonance? It is possible that I have misunderstood the meaning of resonance when wondering how this phenomenon can contribute to caring science in health care. I argue that there is no "or," as stated in the question in this section's heading. As I understand Rosa (2019), resonance is a mode of relationship. He defines resonance as:

> A specifically cognitive, affective, and bodily relationship to the world in which subjects are touched and occasionally even 'shaken' down to the neural level by certain segments of the world, but at the same time are also themselves 'responsively,' actively, and influentially related to the world and experience themselves as effective in it—this is the nature of the responsive relation of 'vibrating wire' between subject and world (2019, p. 163).

Later on, Rosa precisely states that resonance is a mode of relationships: "Hence one of the key hypotheses of this book is that *resonance is not an emotional state, but a mode of relation*" (2019, p. 168). This is interesting and relevant to my present reflections within this section. It led me to wonder whether the encounter I had with the female patient in my example was not dependent on either of our emotions and/or feelings, but rather on how we experienced and acknowledged each other. During this encounter, sovereign and spontaneous life utterances played an important role, from her spontaneous expressions of pain within the trusting encounter, to her openness of speech, and to her act of silently relating her needs to me as a nurse.

As Løgstrup writes in a frequently quoted passage, we, as people, "never have anything to do with each other without taking each other's lives into our hands" (1991, p. 25). This means that each encounter we have, impacts the other person to a varying degree. Small things that happen during an encounter may have a significant impact on how the other individual experiences happiness and success in life (Løgstrup, 1991, p. 25). This is not only an important ethical demand to remember, but a means of respecting our interdependence as humans. This ethical demand requires that I meet the needs of others and do so on my own initiative. As I have previously stated, it is tacit but nevertheless present in encounters between two human beings. At the same time, Løgstrup emphasizes that, within an encounter, my responsibility to the other person does not mean that I should take over their responsibility for themselves. Rather, each person has a responsibility toward themselves that must be respected (1991, p. 39).

In my case, this personal responsibility led me to suggest to the patient that she go for an X-ray and to then listen to her response. In this case, she cried for help, which indicated to me that she was relieved when I suggested taking further action in addition to administering painkillers. However, this was not a straightforward and clear interpretation, but one that that I, along with the nurse assistant, made based on our previous experience with this patient and her expressions in the current situation. In such situations, it is important for nurses to have professional morality, to respect the ethical demands of their position, and to understand how sovereign life utterances play a role in their encounters with patients.

MORAL PRACTICES IN HEALTH CARE PROFESSIONS

Spontaneous life utterances are fundamentally crucial to the moral practices of health professions. To be a professional nurse requires a sense of respect for moral norms and values. Nurses should be aware of the importance of not pursuing self-interest but instead focusing on the interests of the care receiver. It is equally important for nurses to update their knowledge within their health care specialty and to respect confidentiality, as is legally required. This is fundamental for maintaining a patient's trust in their nurse as well as the health care services, they receive. This level of sustained trust is necessary for a patient to feel safe in expressing their vulnerability through sovereign life utterances, and to trust that their vulnerability will be received in a respectful and sympathetic way.

Maintaining professional morality and conducting moral practices are important for several reasons. Among them, I argue, is that this aspect of modernity allows professionals to establish a relationship with their patients, according to the theory of resonance presented by Rosa (2019). Also, this allows nurses and other health care personnel to recognize and fulfill the ethical demand as described by Løgstrup (1991) and further elaborated on by Martinsen (2012). However, Løgstrup warns against claiming that one carries out certain actions to fulfill the ethical demand (1991, p. 123). If someone claims that the ethical demand requires you to act towards the other person through specific and certain actions, one should be suspicious (Løgstrup, 1991, p. 123). As an example, the caregiver may feel compelled to provide assistance that the care receiver would rather decline. The care receiver is then treated as a body-soul-mechanism for the giver rather than as a human being (Løgstrup, 1991, p. 76). The body-soul-mechanism means to treat the patient more like a robot without free will and emotions, rather than treating them with the dignity and autonomy of a unique human being. As Vetlesen (2001) suggests, this is a misunderstanding of both the ethical demand and care ethics.

Hansen (2020) also explores the professional role in a caring relationship. He warns against establishing "professional contact" between the caregiver and the care receiver. This is because caring relies on sovereign life utterances as phenomena one must be in resonance with, which goes beyond establishing "caring relations" (Hansen, 2020). However, the care may be experienced by the care receiver as being acknowledged according to the understanding of caring science as outlined by Martinsen (1991; 2012), which includes a moral aspect as well as relational and practical aspects. Several scholars have noted that interdependence is a central phenomenon in caring relationships (Løgstrup, 1991; Martinsen, 1991; Vetlesen, 2001). Martinsen (1991) points out that according to the moral aspect of caring in the understanding of care ethics, the caregiver should meet the care receivers as human beings. That is, they should be met as persons with autonomy who are, at the same time, part of a collective community in which the caregiver has a responsibility to the vulnerable persons (see also Tronto, 2020). The care receiver is dependent on the caregiver and the relationship is imbalanced, even though both persons have the same human value and are interdependent in the encounter. Vetlesen (2001) argues that caring respects the care receiver's independence by addressing their vulnerability and preventing death. Both Martinsen (1991) and Vetlesen (2001) claim that responsibility for the vulnerable leads individuals to act morally in their daily encounters with one another. These actions are based on care relation characteristics such as power imbalances, ambiguous caring actions, and the fact the evolution of relationships and caring actions often have unforeseeable consequences (Martinsen, 1991; Vetlesen, 2001).

Martinsen (1991) points out that the caregiver should freely provide care based on the understanding that the care receiver is equal in value, even though the caregiver and receiver may not be equal in power. It is essential to establish how health care personnel can and should act within the context of their professional lives to incorporate the elements of resonance, ethical demands, and caring as a moral practice into a field that constantly demands effectiveness, innovation, and self-improvement. However, I argue that resonance and sovereign life utterances go beyond merely adopting moral practices. Rather, these phenomena provide other positive experiences for both patients and nurses during health care encounters.

Martinsen (2012) elaborates on caring as a phenomenon and describes six ethical challenges therein. The first challenge is that all human beings have the same fundamental conditions, such as vulnerability and dependency. Second, taking an ethical approach is paramount when one responds to another person's emergency and has the urge to act. (This challenge is similar to Travelbee's [1971] sympathy phase.) Third, our ethics must be expressed through cultural constructions like norms and rituals. This leads to the fourth challenge, which states that we are limited by temporality. The fifth challenge is that, because of ethical insight, we must respect each other's vulnerability and treat one another with dignity. Finally, the sixth challenge is a caregiver's ability to differentiate between two different forms of taking action: relieving another person's vulnerability and avoiding taking full responsibility for the vulnerable person (Martinsen, 2012, pp. 116–119).

These six ethical challenges are relevant to a caregiver's ability to meet the vulnerable person, the patient, in a resonant and caring way. Due to these challenges, we must have phenomenon-driven care where shared vulnerability is the fundamental meeting point of the health care encounter. When reflecting on my own experience, in a sense, I shared the pain my patient was experiencing when I decided to make a different choice. I felt her pain in my body as a shared phenomenon of vulnerability. I was responding to a call from the spontaneous life utterances of the vulnerable patient. It did not feel like a choice upon which I deliberated, but instead, it was a response to my ethical demand in a resonant human-to-human relationship.

CONCLUSION

To bring this discussion to a logical close, I return to the questions posed in this chapter's introduction: In what ways can an existential and phenomenological research and practice approach with a special focus on the phenomena of wonder, silence, and human flourishing help to re-humanize professionalism and practices in the field of health? And whether vulnerability aligns with the "existential-phenomenological dialogical wondering theory" of this book or whether it raises some challenges? Perhaps the sovereign life utterances phenomena can only be experienced in a resonant way, as an aspect of relationship experienced between two human beings in a special mode of encounter. Rosa writes:

> As we know from everyday experience, the question of whether resonant relationships can actually be established where we expect or anticipate them depends on a multitude of contextual factors and the complex interplay between them. This can sometimes also lead to having resonant experiences where we *least* expect them (1991, p. 382).

I recommend having resonant relationships in nursing and the health care services because if nurses can establish human-to-human relationships with persons in need of care and treatment, that is a quality of service that can be experienced as resonant by the patient and the nurse. It may not be possible to plan to have a resonant relationship where sovereign life utterances play an important role and the caring is morally, practically, and relationally present. Neither should participants in the health care system strive to be resonant and strive to experience sovereign life utterances. As explained throughout this chapter, these phenomena are spontaneous and sovereign. Life utterances are experienced organically in a situation and they cannot be forced to happen. However, these phenomena can only happen if the patient trusts the nurse, experiences compassion and comfort, and can be honest about the vulnerability they are experiencing. The mode of the relationship between the nurse and the care receiver may then become resonant during the encounter. This can even occur spontaneously when resonance is not expected, and the two parties can meet as human beings who acknowledge and respect one another as unique individuals.

Finally, the resonant relationship will have to be an encounter where sovereign life utterances can thrive and be fully experienced because it is a resonant relationship within a caring environment. An increased focus on care ethics in the health care sector can contribute to the humanization of encounters with vulnerable patients in need of assistance, care, and support. Care ethics allow these patients to be met with respect for their status as unique human beings and vulnerable persons. Sovereign life utterances and a resonant relationship can help maintain this dynamic so that patients feel humanized during their health care services and are helped by caregivers to flourish even while experiencing vulnerability.

NOTES

1. I am aware of Patricia Benner's (1994) interpretive phenomenological theory, but in this chapter, I will rely on the traditions of Western-Europe and Nordic countries when discussing existential-phenomenology, as this will open up new dimensions in caring science.
2. Cf. Polanyi's concept of tacit knowledge.

REFERENCES

Benner, P., & Wrubel, J. (1989). *The primacy of caring.* Addison-Wesley Publishing.

Benner, P. (Ed.). (1994). *Interpretive Phenomenology.* Sage Publishing.

Engster, D. (2018). Care ethics, dependency, and vulnerability. *Ethics and Social Welfare, 13*(2), 100–14. https://doi.org/10.1080/17496535.2018.1533029.

Gilligan, C. (1982). *In a different voice: Psychological theory and women's development.* Harvard University Press.

Hansen, F. T. (2020). *Professionel kontakt handler også om at være i takt med det underfulde. (Professional contact is about being in tune with wondering).* Presentation at seminar at Brandbjerg University College, Denmark.

Hansen F. T., & Jørgensen L. B. (2020). A contribution to the ontology of the fundamentals of care framework from a wonder-based approach. *Journal of Clinical Nursing, 29*(1–11), 1797–807. https://doi.org/10.1111/jocn.15272.

Jerak-Zuiderent, S. (2015). Accountability from somewhere and for someone: Relating with care. *Science as Culture, 24*(4), 412–35. https://doi.org/10.1080/09505431.2015.1050368.

Kierkegaard, S. (2013). *Kjerlighedens Gjerninger. (The acts of love).* Gyldendal.

Kittay, E. F. (2020). Vulnerability and the moral nature of dependency relations. In *Love's labor: Essays on women, equality and dependency*. (2nd ed.). (pp. 49–73). Routledge; Taylor & Francis.

Løgstrup, K. E. (1991). *Den etiske fordring. (The ethical demand).* Gyldendal. (Original work published 1956).

Løgstrup, K. E., (2013). *Opgør med Kierkegaard. (Settlement with Kierkegaard).* Aarhus: Forlaget Klim.

Martinsen, K. (1991). *Omsorg, sykepleie og medisin: Historisk-filosofiske essays (Care, nursing and medicine: Historical-philosophical essays).* Tano.

Martinsen, K. (2012). *Løgstrup & Sygeplejen. (Løgstrup & Nursing).* Forlaget KLIM.

Polanyi, M. (2009). *The tacit dimension.* University of Chicago Press. (Original work published 1966).

Rosa, H. (2019). *Resonance: A Sociology of Our Relationship to the World.* Polity Press.

Slettebø, Å. (2012). En fenomenologisk inngang til profesjonsetikken: Tillit i praksis—forutsetning eller fortjeneste? (A phenomenal entrance to professional ethics: Trust in practice—assumption or merit?) *Nordisk sygeplejeforskning, 2*(2), 145–55.

Slettebø, Å., & Fredriksson, L. (2015). The significance of caring. *Scandinavian Journal of Caring Sciences, 29*(2), 203–204. https://doi.org/10.1111/scs.12227.

Travelbee, J. (1963). What do we mean by RAPPORT? *American Journal of Nursing, 63*(2), 70–72. http://dx.doi. org/10.2307/3452595.

Travelbee, J. (1964). What's wrong with sympathy? *American Journal of Nursing, 64*(1), 68–71. http://dx.doi. org/10.2307/3452776.

Travelbee, J. (1971). *Interpersonal aspects of nursing* (2nd ed.). F. A. Davis Company.

Travelbee, J. (2020). *Human-to-human relationship model.* Current Nursing. http://currentnursing.com/nursing_theory/Joyce_Travelbee.html.

Tronto, J.C. (2016). *Protective care or Democratic care? Some reflections on terrorism and care* [Comments prepared for presentation]. SIGNAL, Cifas.

van Nistelrooij, I. & Leget, C. (2016). Against dichotomies: On mature care and self-sacrifice in care ethics. *Nursing ethics, 24*(6), 694–703. https://doi.org/10.1177/0969733015624475.

Vetlesen, A. J. (2001). Omsorg—mellom avhengighet og autonomi. (Care—between dependence and autonomy.) In K. W. Ruyter & A. J. Vetlesen (Eds.), *Omsorgens tvetydighet. (The ambiguity of care)* (pp. 27–40). Gyldendal Akademisk.

Vetlesen, A. J. (2010), Tillitens forrang. (The preference of trust). *Nytt Norsk Tidsskrift, (New Norwegian Journal), 27*(3), 325–29.

Chapter 5

Your Thoughts Don't Have Words Every Day

Poetic Quality and the Health Professions

Merel Visse

Are you too deeply occupied to say if my Verse is alive?

—Emily Dickinson

One day, on a sunny afternoon at the start of my work as a researcher, I met with John, the spouse of Sarah, who had just passed away. I met with him in the context of a responsive evaluation project on palliative care that I carried out with a colleague. One of us reported on this shared endeavor in the past (Abma, 2004). In this chapter I will expand on my experiences as the on-site researcher, and reflect on them from a stance of wonder.

We knew John's wife, Sarah, had cancer of the thyroid and suffered a long sickbed. She was planned to be transferred from the oncology ward of the hospital to a nearby hospice, but suddenly fell too ill to be transported safely. Her admittance to the hospital ward and the relationship between John and the oncology ward nurses were filled with conflict. The nurses referred to him as a "difficult case."

Sitting at John's dining room table, I did attempt to understand what had happened. I 'conducted' my interview to hear his version of what happened. He answered my questions dutifully, generously, but the interview did not flow. Connecting with him was challenging. He was angry, mostly. Angry with the nurses for lack of attention and care for his wife. Angry with a system that did not understand him. His strong emotions were at the foreground. I felt that to a certain extent, they stood in the way of me understanding his experiences so we could learn from them. I sensed there was more to his story than the story of anger that I heard. I thought his account a little too convinced and closed, not 'alive,' despite his passionate voice (or perhaps because of it?).

I learned that most stories that ring true, including this one, are full of paradoxes and polyphonies. Some experiences are just too complex not to be an enigma. Much later, that would become one of my main criteria for knowing whether someone shared something meaningful: I would search for the aliveness, the ambiguity, the personal struggles, and the humanity in their anecdotes. I would learn, too, that my inability to connect with John was not a lack of connection with *him*, but with something else. I was not connected to wonder. Perhaps it was insufficient meta-physical listening and 'being with,' . . . what Heidegger would call "*Befindlichkeit* and *Gelassenheit*" (Hansen, 2012, 8). But back then, when I had just entered the research field, more than twenty-five years ago, when I found myself in that dining room, what I was aware of was his closed posture, his watery eyes, and tensed muscles. Watery, not from sadness, but because of his frustration, not having the missing words.

I sensed that something else was going on. It took me several years to find the words for that. It had something to do with this. During my first visit, just before we sat down, he made tea. The teacups were deliberately chosen ("my best ones"); the kettle was already on when I pressed his bell. He had been expecting me. When he served me the cake he'd bought especially for my coming, his hands trembled. Every gesture seemed to be enacted with anticipation. Perhaps apprehension. "This is not just an interview," I thought, and then, a bit more anxious: "What does he want from me?" I felt a heaviness coming over me.

The clock ticked by. I learned the nature and severity of the conflict with the nurses. The nurses had told me:

> He was with his wife continuously. He was always around. It prevented us from sitting at the bedside to hold her hand. It made it impossible for me to develop a relationship with her. She needed a lot of care and he had to learn everything from us. He wanted to learn these things. In the end, when he knew everything that we could teach him, it was as if he turned around and said 'I know everything about my wife and you know nothing.' It was very disappointing—especially if you want to help someone.

The nurses assumed that his anger partly stemmed from the deep grief about his wife's death, but they seemed to be open to learn from what happened too. Hearing about his experiences made them wonder, what is 'good' palliative care?

Gradually, perhaps after an hour, I sensed a change in his mood. It was as if we were moving to a space beyond his anger. There were small but significant remarks that captured something of his experience. For example that he felt a need to be seen, for his wife to be seen. And that beyond his disappointment was deep sadness and powerlessness. That he experienced renewed hope after finding better words for his experiences ('The writing is the last thing I did for Sarah. I owed it to her. I cannot do anything for her anymore, but hopefully, other people can benefit from it'). In hindsight, my interview grew from getting information to *having a personal conversation.* And perhaps even beyond that, but I will move to that soon.

After that first encounter, I went back several times to his house to continue the dialogue. Every time I would bring a text that I had written. A poetic text. Gradually his experiences were captured. My colleague and I agreed that poetry can provide us a glimpse into an experiential world often unseen and unacknowledged. Whether conventional poetry or jotting down poetic thoughts, it invites the 'potential of caring' (Hamington & Rosenow, 2019, p.2; Tobia, 2020). So: we wrote a poem. Together. Our poem was meant to evoke something in a hypothetical reader. I had the nurses in mind as primary readers. Here is one stanza:

> Sarah was a difficult case
> Never before they experienced a case like her.
> But this 'difficult case'
> happened to be my wife!!
> *there is no cure for this cancer*
> She became weaker and weaker.
> And then she couldn't breathe anymore.
> She was choking, She was dying.

Day and night, he was at her side. The nurses did not have to do anything. He did it all. That is how he felt. But he felt unseen by the nurses: *They did not see me anymore.* Simultaneously, he felt he had to be his wife's guardian—*to be on watch continuously, so that the nurses 'would not hurt her.'* Would not hurt her.

Our study and his poem became a vehicle for dialogue between the nurses and the man about what constitutes 'good palliative care.'

In another publication I reported on my role as a facilitator in that study (Visse et al., 2012). In that publication, I wanted to learn about what it meant for me to be an evaluator of palliative care. Should I also want to be a facilitator and advocate? I wondered. Although they overlap, I decided against advocate, as that would limit my perspective to a singular perspective, instead of being open to other interpretations of the nurses and other health professionals. I favored the role of facilitator: this provided me with the space to explore connections between the perspectives of John and the nurses.

That day, though, sitting at his table, I did not think about those roles at all. Instead, I found myself caring. Paying attention, being receptive, wanting to hear what he tried to express but was incapable of expressing. Research is not care. But I do believe that a caring stance evokes insights that a detached approach does not. A caring stance may capture complexity and depth. Not because of empathy, nor because of identification. There is a fine balance between over- or under-identification and being able to truly listen to and being receptive to your respondents (Visse et al., 2012). At that moment, in that dining room, I learned about what it takes to be a good researcher, and that it also entails the art of listening and seeing from an ontological and pre-ontological wonder. But at the time, I was not aware of these insights yet. In hindsight, I may have sensed an ethical demand that I could not ignore, although I did not know what the demand was (Løgstrup, 1997). That would unfold with time. Sitting there, sipping my tea and listening to his story, I may have detected that demand, intuitively. As if—again: this is me speaking in hindsight—just 'gathering knowledge' would be immoral and dehumanizing. "Knowledge production" was and still are magic words in academia. The word 'production' may be misleading, as the anthropologist Barbara Myerhoff already addressed in 1978. What was I concerned about?

Today I am concerned because I know that "our thoughts don't have words every day," to quote Emily Dickinson. Many of my thoughts do not. Many thoughts never become words. Perhaps there are no thoughts without words at all. Would there be images instead, I wonder? Can we think without words at all? Some say there is a close connection between images and thinking conceptually. It is not only language that plays the communicative role in our understanding of the world around us. Thinking has indeed been thought of vocalizing, and thought and language are inseparable. But this belief is limited. A child that cannot think or imagine before it is unable to speak? Anyone who lives with a child knows how inquisitive a child can be. A child who cannot think or imagine, cannot survive (Eisner, 1978). Cognitive growth and reasoning are closely connected to developing one's perception. Sensory perception is paramount to the ability to reason well about concepts. Without imagination there is no concept. Eliot Eisner, the well-known art educator, argued the poetic imagination probably comes closest to the most sophisticated forms of cognition (1992). Poetic imagination is 'extra-logical'; the meanings conveyed can be seen as the product of human rationality that goes beyond reasoning.

In any case, perhaps the articulation of the words may take a while. Words need time to unfold. Can we 'tease them out'? A constructivist would say: the words did not exist with the thoughts, there to be unfolded, but were formed by the speaker. He would say, not as the thought itself but as an expression stimulated by the thoughts. I will get back to that thought soon.

First, I take a short detour to explore what my interest in 'expression' has to do with how we view knowledge production in academia and health care. No matter how words come into existence, in academia and medicine we seldom have the time to listen to thoughts, and to a pre-linguistic realm of our experience. We need to 'produce knowledge' as fast and with as little expense as possible. Systemic pressures do not do justice to the complexities of the experiences of the people we work with. From our participants to our clients and other stakeholders. The meanings of "gathering data" are complex. Along my research, I became interested in another view of what it means to 'gather data.' I was ready for an approach that honors existential, ontological, and pre-linguistic dimensions of our world. An approach that centers around contemplation, attentiveness, and care. An approach that resists the economic priority of knowledge production. One that is open to dimensions that are verbal, and non-verbal as well. That is what my work with Finn Hansen and Carlo Leget became about (Visse, Hansen & Leget, 2019, 2020)

Years after that first study on palliative care (way back in 1996), in another article, I would argue for viewing research as a *praxis of care* (Visse & Niemeijer, 2017). And more recently, Bob Stake and I thought about a *paradigm of care* (Stake & Visse, 2020). With the editors of this book, Finn and Carlo, I wrote about *apophatic inquiry* (Visse, Hansen, Leget, 2020). Apophatic inquiry is about "thinking questioningly" (Findlay, 2002, p. 66, citing Patočka, 2002), focusing on "truth experiences" (Gadamer, 1960/1975) and phenomenality or life itself as the heart of inquiry.

In all these texts, my view is that having interviews, being in conversations with respondents or participants in a case, observing them living their lives, is part of a *caring* relationship. It is not part of a relationship of appropriation: where we instrumentally meet with respondents to 'get data.' Qualitative, phenomenological health research can only work if we put ourselves on the line too. Just like our respondents. Showing the willingness to engage, genuinely and open. Being open not solely for the scaling dimensions of the world, but also for ontological ones, cherishing *living understandings* (Risser, 2019). Hans-Georg Gadamer, the German philosopher and former student of Martin Heidegger, once wrote:

> In human relations the important thing is, as we have seen, to experience the Thou truly as a Thou—i.e., not to overlook his claim but to let him really say something to us. Here is where openness belongs. But ultimately this openness

> does not exist only for the person who speaks; rather, anyone who listens is fundamentally open. Without such openness to one another there is no genuine human bond. Belonging together always also means being able to listen to one another. When two people understand each other, this does not mean that one person "understands" the other. Similarly, "to hear and obey someone" (auf jemanden horen) does not mean simply that we do blindly what the other desires. We call such a person slavish (horig). Openness to the other, then, involves recognizing that I myself must accept some things that are against me, even though no one else forces me to do so (Gadamer, 1975, 390).

FALLING INTO CONVERSATION

One challenge in understanding someone's lifeworld is to invite someone to *express* what occurred. Conveying thoughts, feelings, intuitions in a conversation is about experiencing "the coming into language of the thing itself" (Gadamer, 1975, 371). Gadamer wrote that expressing is not a will-full act. On the contrary. Ideally, the 'real' conversation is never one we were planning nor prepared to have. We "fall" into a conversation (ibid, 385). The conversation is shaped by our readiness for it, and by the Other's readiness, by what was said before, by what language is available, and certainly by the context. We fall into a particular conversation, however planned, largely by chance, hewing loose boundaries, flying off on tangents.

A conversation on the experiences of anger, such as in the example above, was needed, would be valued, but it left out something important at its very start. That conversation, anchored in disappointment and hurt, prevented us from going to a space of serious wonder, of entering the "deeper ontological ground, which we trust without knowing why" (Hansen, 2012, 11). For him to share his lived experiences, he needed to let his story about anger and blame go (for a while), and move to other dimensions of his inner world. This asks for a "not-expecting-to-know" attitude (ibid). According to Gadamer, the process of understanding starts when we experience a break-down (Gadamer, 1975, p. 160; Gadamer, 2004, p. 182). The need for understanding arises when we experience something which 'interrupts the ordinary, taken for granted aspects of existence' (McManus Holroyd, 2007, p. 2). When something happens that we do not expect, or someone gives an answer which is not in line with our preconceived ideas, our view of the world is challenged, and the question of meaning comes to the fore. How can we make sense of the strange event or response? As long as the situation is familiar, events are experienced within a natural frame of meaning.

When we are confronted with something unfamiliar, such as an illness, we experience a tension between the unfamiliar and the familiar. Illness is an example of an experience that is likely to cause tension between ourselves and the world. The hermeneutic task is not hiding this tension, not attempting assimilation, but, Gadamer argues, by 'consciously bringing it out' (1975, p. 273). Dissolving the tension between what is strange and familiar is one of the characteristics of the process of understanding. When working on this chapter, my colleague Finn Hansen wondered whether this is true. He wrote: "when feeling in resonance with a living mystery, do I then 'understand' this? No, I do though, understand, acknowledge that I am in touch with something wonderful, or enigmatic, which I have to/or become aware of with reverence. But this kind of 'understanding' (understanding as an awareness of a resonance with something enigmatic and living) is not, in my view, a dissolving of the tension between what is strange (enigmatic) and familiar. On the contary, this kind of understanding helps me to respect and keep the differences and mystery alive. Or, maybe better said, "to see the familiar with or from the light of the mystery." I was thankful for this comment and I mainly agree with him, but there may still be instances when understanding does involve the dissolution of tension. I wonder if w eshould distinguish different types of situations and understandings. Perhaps it largely depends on how we, if we take an example such as illness, view the nature of illness. Illness can be interpreted as a consequence of disturbance of natural processes (either in the classical sense of a disturbance of body fluids, or more modern, as a disturbance in organ functioning), or as a consequence of improper behavior (either in the classical sense of a sin against God's commands, or in the modern sense of unhealthy behavior, such as smoking). When making sense of why we got ill, we can search for explanations that match these categories. Our illness can either be caused by the disturbance of a natural process or/and by a consequence of improper behavior. When we cannot find a connection between one these reasons, we may not being able to understand why we got ill. Then, all we have is a mystery. We are beyond understanding why something in our lives unfolded in a particular way. Accepting this mystery may also be seen as a form of understanding, but an understanding not as in interpretation, but as in accepting.

According to Gadamer, this would relate to a subtle process of widening one's perspective, to include the mystical. This is a dialogical process. Does this also mean that entering a space of wonder is always dialogical? It is perhaps best through dialogue that we foster a needed 'not-expecting-to-know' attitude and becoming attuned to the mood of ourselves and others. This does not only happen intentionally but occurs in and through the naturality of conversation. Therefore, creating spaces where we can wonder together, or with ourselves, spaces where we can live the hermeneutic process and be open to lived experiences, becomes valued.

Going back to the field of research, being a good researcher means caring. I mark my interviews 'good' when I sense the presence of a relationship with the other from which a meaningful conversation can unfold. Together we move through a hermeneutic quest. Together we can wonder and search to listen to the phenomena that present themselves. Sometimes by interpretation, other times by accepting mysteries. That is not simple. I find that hard. What is meant by this 'hermeneutic quest,' how we listen, question, and support others and ourselves in expressing their and our inner world? What to do when we find it impossible to express what's inside, when words are inadequate? How do we hear and express ourselves not only from the ontic realms of our existence, but also from the (pre)ontological and apophatic dimensions of our experience and thinking. We turn to Gadamer again:

> Just as things, those units of our experience of the world that are constituted by their suitability and their significance, are brought into language, so the tradition that has come down to us is again brought to speak in our understanding and interpretation of it. The linguistic nature of this bringing into language is the same as that of the human experience of the world in general. This is what has finally led our analysis of the hermeneutical phenomenon to the discussion of the relationship between language and world (Gadamer, 1975, 452).

Gadamer called our unexpressed and inexpressible thoughts: the *verbum interium* (the inner word). To him, the words we say, the language that comes out of our mouth, are closely connected with our inner thought. He spoke about an "intimate unity of thought and speech" (Arthos, 2009, 6). This may explain why, when we do succeed in finding the words for our experiences, when we are able to tell the doctor what is going on inside, there may be release, resolution. Meaning, maybe. Even joy, sometimes. But this is rarely a solitary act, something done by individuals alone, he says. The dialogue is so greatly needed, Gadamer argued. I wonder if the dialogue is so paramount indeed. I wonder if this goes against Emily Dickinson's line on thoughts not having words every day. I wonder if there is an unbreachable gulf. I wonder if a dialogue, a conversation, is able to tease the words out. Again, expressing is not a will-full act, Gadamer said. The words cannot be captured intact, and they are also not like approximations in language that get closer to our experiences than what so far is expressed. And although poetry may go at experience indirectly, circling the issue, turning up clues that allow new interpretations, it is not a plaster to find the right words.

TESTING THE GIFT OF LANGUAGE

So, here you move quite fast, Hans-Georg. Let's take a closer at this. Yes, indeed: some phenomena, some mental traffic patterns, test the aptitudes of our language. They show us that verbal expression, finding the right words, may defy us. Saying it in words may be more than challenging, it may be impossible. Pain is one of those phenomena. We all know it is difficult to express pain or hurt, physical, mental, spiritual, and emotional. Elaine Scarry, in her book, *The Body in Pain*, wrote that "to have great pain is to have certainty; to hear that another person has pain is to have doubt" (Scarry, 1985, p. 4). She says, "Physical pain not only resists language, but actively destroys it. It resists objectification in language" (ibid). Images or poetic language may assist us to tell the doctor or nurse what we are experiencing, and which story our pain is part of, if there is such a story. But still, nothing can really express the pain as we feel it. This reminds me of a poem that Emily Dickinson (1830–1886) wrote. It is titled 'the mystery of pain':

> Pain has an element of blank;
> It cannot recollect
> When it began, or if there were
> A day when it was not.
> It has no future but itself,
> Its infinite realms contain
> Its past, enlightened to perceive
> New periods of pain[1]

'Its infinite realms contain': this points toward the vastness of the experience of pain. Many experiences and thoughts are "more immediate, more enigmatic, more complex, more nuanced, and more ambitious than any description can do justice to" (Van Manen, 2014, p. 242). Writers, artist, spouses, friends: not all the time, but sometimes, they all search for ways to express their inner thoughts. Some inner worlds, and worlds within worlds, are rich and large, much larger than that outside them. Others are less deep. But all are profound in their humanity. There are thoughts and phenomena that are hard to express. Even though we may be able to perceive them, once we think we have captured them, we may lose them. Perhaps these kinds of thoughts take more time to come to the foreground, to surface. Artists are aware as no-one else. Emily Dickinson seemed to know it when she wrote:

> Perception of an object costs
> Precise the Object's loss —
> Perception in itself a Gain
> Replying to its Price —

The Object Absolute — is nought —
Perception sets it fair
And then upbraids a Perfectness
That situates so far — [2]

With Emily, many philosophers grasp the limits of language. Socrates argued that "we can never understand justice if we do not live it. Justice, like every authentic reality, is indefinable" (Hansen quoting Hadot, 2012, p. 13). *Living* understandings was also part of Gadamer's perspective on language. He understood that the difficulty with expressing our thoughts is not an error in our language, but is a powerful feature of it, and perhaps even a requirement for words to 'incarnate,' even though they never fully will. No speech gets close, he would say, and "yet, this is the enigma," my colleague Finn Hansen responded when he read a previous version of this chapter. Our words need time to unfold from an ontological realm into the realm of practical discourse. Gadamer:

> The occasionality of human speech is not a casual imperfection of its expressive power; it is, rather, the logical expression of the living virtuality of speech that brings a totality of meaning into play, without being able to express it totally. (Gadamer, 1975, 454)

Hansen interpreted Gadamer's notion of the balance or tension needed between the phenomenological and the dialectical, calling them the "lyrical impulse and the Socratic impulse" (Hansen, 2012, 13). Both the phenomenological sense of our intuitions, feelings and moods (the 'lyrical impulses'), and our existential dialectical and critical questioning dialogue (the 'Socratic impulses') are needed in order to access lived experience through language. But it is not enough. In order for us to connect with the ontological, the pre-linguistic, we need wonder: "in wonder we transcend our language and get in touch with the world in a way that brings new life to the words we use to express the impression life makes on us" (2012, 14). When we connect with that which we are not able to express, we can be in wonder and "witness a 'world-ing'; that is, a world that is coming to be here-and-now" (ibid). Wonder provides the balance between the lyrical and Socratic impulse.

EMILY DICKINSON AS A PHENOMENOLOGIST

Emily Dickinson has shown how to approach language in a way that honors the process of unfolding, and of the presence of a realm that is indefinable. In her poetry she *does* what Hans-Georg Gadamer wrote about: she explores the relationship between our thoughts and our expressions.

Usually, language is cognitive; it tends to intellectualize our awareness and experience. It is also an expressive medium. When, in our research, we write to evoke a response, language is about expression of "the objects to come into words" (Gadamer, 1975, 390). Gadamer used the word 'objects' but he seemed to refer to the Thou, not to It. Narratives and anecdotes that are written to evoke a conversation with the reader, move beyond the cognitive function of language. They aim for a relationship with the reader. The reader gets a glimpse of the inner word as expressed on paper. Gadamer said:

> Thus the hermeneutical phenomenon proves to be a special case of the general relationship between thinking and speaking, whose enigmatic intimacy conceals the role of language in thought. (Gadamer, 1975, 390)

In response to reading this chapter, Finn wrote to me: "What is said here? What is meant by thought here, is, I think, the thoughts that come out of 'thinking.' But not thinking as reflecting, but thinking as medtative contemplation. One cannot 'think' without beein in deep wonder *and* resonance with a living mystery, as in the phenomenon in and by it self."

Dickinson enacted the world not through objective analysis of the world, not through trying to access phenomena—such as in the phenomenology of Husserl—but through the *unfolding of language,* as mentioned above. She was deeply interested in concepts beyond human understanding, such as divinity, pain, death. Her work is contemplative and individual, but always an invitation to engage with a reader. As a wordsmith, a writer, she did not focus on publication, but endlessly worked on improving her poems, across her lifetime. I turned toward her poems, and toward scholars who wrote about her approach, because I found her approach meaningful for research on lived experiences. I also recognize her lack of interest in publication, but in working on texts. For me: having a deadline works contrary to the space that I need to listen, to let insights unfold at their own pace. I also resonate with Emily's interest in what was beyond the empirical. By meandering around everyday ordinary experiences, she examined what they strived to say without naming them directly. By doing so, she shows us the 'world-ing' (Hansen, 2012,14) of a phenomenon. Not capturing it but making us a witness of its birth.

Meandering around a Thou, or an experience can be seen as an aesthetic quality (Franke, 2007). Dickenson played with the limits of language and reached out to inarticulate experiences such as suffering, hope, loss, and love, experiences that have significant meaning in medicine and care. Such inarticulates may sound vague or otherworldly, but there is virtue in vagueness. Dickinson does not want to draw us away from reality into an imaginary world necessarily, but she does draw us deeper into an inquirying world for sure. I find her poetry utterly realist. It shows what Gadamer mentioned about the importance of both: on the one hand the discursive realm of life, and on the other hand, the existential dimension of life.

> . . . one word that we say to one another and that is said to us (theologically, "the" Word of God)—but the unity of this word, as we saw, always unfolds step by step in articulated discourse. (Gadamer, 1975, 454)

Here, Gadamer means the words that are spoken, articulated, are not articulated at the moment they are said. We hear them, yes, but their 'unity' needs to unfold, step by step, with time.

Dickinson had an eye for the flux of experience, for consciousness, for existential phenomena such as time, space and mood. Her discourse inquires what it means to be human and how to *live* one's questions through poetry. She was able to 'depict complex bodily states' (Delchamps, 2019, 106). For example this poem about breath and lungs:

> I breathed enough to take the Trick —
> And now, removed from Air —
> I simulate the Breath, so well —
> That One, to be quite sure —
> The Lungs are stirless — must descend
> Among the cunning cells —
> And touch the Pantomime — Himself,
> How numb, the Bellows feels![3]

Her poetry is phenomenological as it leans into pre-linguistic experience that can only partially be known. Despite this fascination with everyday concrete experiences, Dickinson's poetry examines both the 'real' and the 'imaginary.' Yet, not so much to split apart the 'real' and the 'imaginary.' We need both to examine critically. Let's look at this quite famous example by Merleau-Ponty (1968): a mental patient complains that there is talcum powder on her bed. There is no empirical ('real') talcum powder on her bed: it could not be found in sensory reality. The talcum powder is "only in the woman's head," or, as Flannery who discusses this example states, it is "only in her imagination." But if the talcum powder is "only" in the woman's head, or "only" in her imagination, would the powder not still be real? Perhaps the talcum powder in this woman's head is as real as any shaked from a can (Merleau-Ponty, 1968). Our brain may accept both empirical data and phenomenal data as equally real. But there is no need to argue equality in this context (Stake, personal communication). In this example, the medical scientist seems to do most of the talking, perceiving the real as the objective world, that can be tested, whilst the imagination is perceived as a subjective world. I wonder how an existential phenomenolist would talk about the 'real' and 'imagination.'

DASHES AND CAPITALS

Dickinson's poetry is not just poetry. It is poetics. Poetics as an approach favoring indirect ways of knowing, unknowing, and being. A praxis of radical integration of art and life (Arthos, 2013, loc 134 [Kindle Ed]). Dickinson is well known for her play with punctuation and format to induce moments of silence and space. Paying attention to these moments, instead of only textual content, is important too. Perhaps even more important, some would argue. For example, Hansen writes: "it is not what the interlocutors in a Socratic dialogue explicitly express in clear words, strong arguments and consistent concepts and definitions that should catch our attention but rather the silence, hesitation, reluctance, prudence, slowness, openness and listening attitude as well as the truth seeking passion, love, playfulness, humor, and of course, the wonder that follows the words or pauses between the words" (2012, 13). Dickinson *shows* us what white space can say. She is able to destabilize the relationship between language and consciousness. Here is a poem worth a close look:

There is a Languor of the Life
More imminent than Pain —
'Tis Pain's Successor —
When the Soul Has suffered all it can —
A Drowsiness — diffuses —
A Dimness like a Fog
Envelops Consciousness —
As Mists — obliterate a Crag.
The Surgeon — does not
blanch — at pain —
His Habit — is severe —
But tell him that it ceased to feel —
The Creature lying there —
And he will tell you — skill is late —
A Mightier than He —
Has ministered before Him —
There's no Vitality.[4]

And:

Surgeons must be very careful
When they take the knife!
Underneath their fine incisions
Stirs the Culprit — Life![5]

In these poems Dickinson takes an integral approach to pain, expresses its extreme experience, and opposes it with a surgeon's approach to pain: he does not 'blanch': he does not seem to resonate with the pain, unable to respond to it. Did he 'cease' to feel, or is that his habit that ceases to feel the 'creature lying there'? This poem first shows us the differences in experiences of pain, and how complex these differences are. Next, the poem is full of visual features such as dashes, capitals, and punctuation marks—uncommon tools. Dickinson does this on purpose. It is as if she does not allow us to read through the poem in one burst, but wants us to pause, pay attention, guide us. Eliza New, professor of American literature at Harvard, says Dickinson's poems are on the verge of verbal art and visual art. Some call it concrete poetry. William Carlos Williams, for example, does it. The use of capitals gives some words a 'hyperfocus,' something like the fourth wall in a theatre play. "When we capitalize something, it gains on the one hand, an abstractness, a formality. It is sometimes an object. An inhuman, inanimate object given a capital begins to seem more human" (Elisa New, transcript EdX Course on the Poetry of Emily Dickinson). The Pain. The Drowsiness. It gives the experience a humaneness.

Then, the dashes. There are longer ones, and shorter ones. In a talk, Elisa New wonders about the meaning of Dickinson's architectural/visual typography: "Many critics wrote about Dickinson's dashes. Are they pauses, grammatical pauses, pauses of breathing, pauses of feeling, relaxation or tension? Some say they are stitches of pain, doors that need to be opened? Do they open, scarlike"?[6] For the purpose of this chapter, we do not need to know the answer. Wondering about what they are and what they evoke, is part of the ongoing work.

Through Dickinson's words, we access thoughts and experiences. They move us or elevate us in sensory ways, they evoke more thoughts. For example, when we feel strong emotions, sensing a need for a response. Something (be)comes more within reach. But not just her poetry making us access the conversation's thoughts and senses; it is our sensing and thoughts that *emerge through* facing a poetic *quality* (Nancy, 2006, 3). Perhaps this is an 'aliveness' (Weber, 2019), perhaps it is something else, but it 'moves' us, in a way. This 'access' to what moves us is a summons. It is challenging and demands effort. If it were not difficult, we would not be granted access, not be moved by the words, nothing would happen (Nancy & Sparks, 2013, 4). Was this what I felt when I started the interview with John, Sarah's husband? I did not feel moved when he began telling me his story. We needed time to arrive at something meaningful, but it took me multiple conversations and writings. I needed to make an effort. Not an effort that focused on 'producing' or 'making,' but effortless effort, almost. Patience. Waiting. With spaces of silence.

SOME LAST UNCRYSTALLIZED THOUGHTS

Writing and reading are humanistic endeavors. Writing, sharing, and discussing poetry in health contexts is common practice nowadays. In the United States, health and medical humanists encourage poetry written and read by health professionals in hospitals, medical and nursing schools, nursing homes, and the houses of those who live with illness and disability. This chapter adds to those experiences by showing what it means to wonder about an aesthetical approach to language. In this chapter, I hope to have shown you a glimpse of why the aesthetic experience is an indispensable human happening that cannot be attained through other experiences. And why it needs to be honored in its own right. This type of experience is not just a pleasure, but essential to understand what is of meaning to us, to health professionals, to patients and their loved ones. Aesthetic experience—a multi-sensory, aspirational experience—is as pervasive as cognitive activity and practical routine. My work explores how we can infuse discursive approaches with this so meaningful a realm of our experience. Sometimes poetry fosters such an experience of understanding and insight. Other times poetry assist us in connecting with moral intuitions. Researchers and scholars in the field of arts-based research and the humanities know this. They argue for a view of research that is attentive to aesthetic experiences of the people and contexts we aim to understand. In this view, the arts and poetry, but philosophy too, are not being used mechanically, instrumentally, in a utilitarian way to "produce" knowledge or insight. Instead, they invite us to *connect* with our aesthetic experience. This invitation is extended in our publication, "Apophatic Inquiry, living the questions themselves," where we propose a view that invites space for aesthetic consciousness in qualitative inquiry (Visse, Hansen, Leget, 2020). This approach requires us to being humble, to open ourselves to reception, to surrender to the process of insights unfolding. This is of meaning to qualitative researchers and all those who care for others. Because by this, indirectly, we re-imagined the researcher and the health professional as a human being who is more than merely a rational agent, in charge, self-assertive as in early renaissance humanist traditions. Instead, we intend a contemporary humanism—a post-humanism perhaps, and a phenomenology for sure—that decenters the human being as an entangled being. Entangled with the environment, nature, materialities, and a realm we can never fully know.

My students grapple with it every day, and I still do too. We want to serve doctors, nurses, and other health professionals by giving them access to patient's experiences. Learning about the experiences of families, and their own experiences. Recently, I taught a class for medical residents and asked about their biggest concern. One of them said, referring to their role as an essential worker during COVID-19: "Who will pick us up when we get ill?" The silence that fell was significant. A few months ago, I attended a session at one of the local hospitals in New Jersey, Overlook Medical Center in Summit, with a poet-in-residence. I found myself in a room with twenty-five professionals, chaplains, physicians, nurses, health administrators, ethicists, all writing and listening to poetry. Something happened in that room. Something meaningful: writing and listening to poetry gave us a sense of community, the sensus communis, as Gadamer phrases it so aptly, a common way of being, a shared sense of wonder.

Words help us address who we are as entangled human beings. Entangled as in our embeddedness in the institutional, ecological and political realities of hospitals and communities, making these realities and imagining how else they could be. Lyrical and wondrous words connect us with realms of human experience that we cannot know, that are and perhaps remain unseen. Here, the role of our poetic imagination is vital. It helps us to learn about ourselves and others. For health professionals and patients, for all of us, the realm of the unknown is challenging, well beyond the edges of the known. Our society does not reward non-knowing. We deem it is better to know, to exert a sense of (epistemological) control upon our world. But in situations, such as when we care for someone with an illness or disability, we find ourselves in the land of limbo (Levine, 2014, 1). An uncertain and often confined place unfamiliar. There is no map for guidance. The world of poetry, the writing of it, and the exchange about it may connect our immediate experience, "more simple, sensuous and passionate" than philosophy or science (Frye quoting Milton, 1964, 28). This is a little deceiving because it makes us see the sciences as rational, and poetry emotional or connected with the existential realms of experience, but that is not necessarily so. Science, referring to the natural sciences, can be passionate, and the humanities, such as philosophy, the visual arts and poetry can be written from an intellectual stance. Both can make us think about philosophical concepts, and both can show us that philosophizing is so much more than dwelling on philosophical concepts and arguments solely. Dickinson's work illustrated it.

Reading and writing poetry can create a communicative space for creativity and critique. Health professionals and researchers need these spaces with people whose lives are upset, whose thoughts find few words and listeners. It may facilitate a temporary void: a space for health professionals to withdraw from the complexities and challenges and professional jargon of their work, but without isolating them from that reality. Being together, or alone, in such a poetic space, can be an act of resistance. It may be an act of hope too. The hope that our readings touch one another, shed light on something that matters to us, and perhaps to others. Even when:

> Your thoughts don't have words every day
> They come a single time
> Like signal esoteric sips
> Of the communion Wine
> Which while you taste so native seems
> So easy so to be
> You cannot comprehend its price
> Nor its infrequency[7]

ACKNOWLEDGMENTS

Several people read and commented on drafts. I want to thank Bob for helping me to find better wor(l)ds; Liora for our ongoing conversation on the arts; and Finn and Carlo for the quest on the apophatic.

NOTES

1. Dickinson, 1896, poem 19. Emily Dickinson Archive. http://www.edickinson.org.
2. No. 1071, Emily Dickinson Archive. http://www.edickinson.org.
3. No F308A, Emily Dickinson Archive. https://www.edickinson.org/editions/1/image_sets/235560.
4. *The Poems of Emily Dickinson*. Ed. R. W. Franklin. 3 vols. Harvard UP, 1998. Poem number 522A.
5. No F156A: https://www.edickinson.org/editions/1/image_sets/235402.
6. Elisa New, transcript EdX Course on the Poetry of Emily Dickinson.
7. Emily Dickinson, No. 1451. Emily Dickinson Archive. http://www.edickinson.org.

REFERENCES

Abma, T.A. (2004). A difficult relationship between oncology ward staff and a patient's husband: a case study. *International Journal of Palliative Nursing, 10(4)*, 180–84. doi:10.12968/ijpn.2004.10.4.12795.

Arthos, J. (2019). *The Inner Word in Gadamer's Hermeneutics*. Notre Dame: University of Notre Dame Press.

Delchamps, V. (2019). "The Names of Sickness": Emily Dickinson, Diagnostic Reading, and Articulating Disability. *The Emily Dickinson Journal* (28) 2: 106–13.

Dickenson, E. (1896). *The Poems of Emily Dickinson: Series One.* Boston, MA: Roberts Brothers.
Eisner, Eliot (1978). The Impoverished Mind. *Educational Leadership*, 615–23.
Eisner, Eliot (1992). The Misunderstood Role of the Arts in Human Development. *Phi Delta Kappa International* (73)8, pp. 592–93.
Findlay, E. F. (2002). *Caring for the soul in a postmodern age. Politics and phenomenology in the thought of jan patočka.* New York: State University of New York Press.
Franke, W. (2007). *On what cannot be said. Apopathic Discourses in Philosophy, Religion, Literature and the Arts.* Volume 1. Classic Formulations. University of Notre Dame Press, Indiana.
Frye, N. (1964). *The Educated Imagination.* Bloomington: Indiana.
Gadamer, H.-G. (1960/1975): *Truth and Method.* (J. Weinsheimer & D.G. Marshall, Translators). New York/London: Continuum Books.
Gadamer, H.-G. (2004). *Truth and Method.* Continuum, London.
Hamington, M., Rosenow, C. (2019). *Care Ethics and Poetry.* Switzerland: Palgrave.
Hansen, F.T. (2012). One Step Further: The Dance between Poetic Dwelling and Socratic Wonder in Phenomenological Research, *Indo-Pacific Journal of Phenomenology*, (12)2, 1–20.
Levine, C. (2014). *Living in the Land of Limbo: Fiction and Poetry about Family Caregiving.* Nashville: Vanderbilt University Press.
Løgstrop, K.E. (1997). *The Ethical Demand.* Indiana: University of Notre Dame Press.
Merleau-Ponty, M. (1968). *The Visible and the Invisible.* Northwestern University Press, Illinois, USA.
MacManus Holroyd, A.E. (2007). Interpretive Hermeneutic Phenomenology: Clarifying understanding. *Indo-pacific Journal of Phenomenology* (7) 2:1–12.
Manen, M. van (2014). *Phenomenology of Practice.* New York: Routledge.
Myerhoff, B. (1978). *Number our days.* New York: Touchstone.
Nancy, J. (2006). *Multiple arts: The muses II* (S. Sparks, Ed.). Stanford, CA: Stanford University Press, (Risser, 2019).
Scarry, E. (1985). *The Body in Pain: The Making and Unmaking of the World.* New York: Oxford University Press.
Stake, R.E., Visse, M.A. (Fall 2020). *A Care Paradigm.* Charlotte: IAP Publishers.
Tobia, S. (2020). Poetry: a healing voice for the frail and elderly. *Journal of Poetry Therapy,* DOI: 10.1080/08893675.2020.1730598.
Visse, M.A., Hansen, F., Leget, C. (2020). Apophatic Inquiry: How to Live the Questions Themselves. *International Journal of Qualitative Methods,* https://doi.org/10.1177/1609406920958975.
Visse, M.A., Hansen, F., Leget, C. (2019). Visse, M., Hansen, F., Leget, C. (2019). The Unsayable in Arts-Based Research: on the Praxis of Life Itself. *International Journal for Qualitative Methods.* https://doi.org/10.1177/1609406919851392.
Visse, M.A., Abma, T.A., Widdershoven, G.A.M. (2012). Relational responsibilities in responsive evaluation. *Evaluation and Program Planning,* 35(1): 97–104.

Chapter 6

The Call in Nursing

A Silent and Vibrant Place for Human Flourishing

Sine Maria Herholdt-Lomholdt

We are called beyond being
by what have no need of us,
convened to an unknown feast
by a word we cannot utter
(Davenport, 2004, p. xv)

AN EARLY MORNING: A LIVED-EXPERIENCE DESCRIPTION, WRITTEN BY THE NURSE SOPHIA

A pause comes to existence again . . . and silence.

My head is in turmoil . . . I sense powerlessness.

Once again, I have an experience of meeting a relative who has been neglected and put out of action. I would so much like to reach her. I would so much like to give her another experience.

I look at her pale and tired face and ask her if she has been up all night. She confirms it with a 'yes' while she silently nods and looks at a point behind me.

Silence again.

I choose to tell her what I have planned to do: to serve her and her mother breakfast. I also tell her that she can stay with her mother at all times. We will consider her as co-hospitalised.

I tell her that we will offer her coffee and other stuff she needs, and I suggest finding her a bed.

She looks as if it would be nice to get rest.

I further suggest bringing her some towels in case she wants to refresh herself . . . or maybe she would prefer to go home for a while?

She prefers to stay, but a towel would be nice . . . and maybe a toothbrush and a hairbrush as well, she says. I nod and notice her shoulders falling a bit.

She looks as if she evaluates me. Actually, she looks a bit sceptical.

I tell her that she is more than welcome to participate in the care-activities around her mother, as she has been next to her mother all the way through. I also tell her that I would love to help with the things she might find difficult.

I have a peculiar feeling.

A feeling that it is impossible for me to get up from the chair!

Something is on its way . . . I have no idea of what it is.

Silence . . . ?

I sense I should be quiet . . .

I should certainly not be superficial.

I have a feeling that she has something on her mind . . .

The daughter looks at me. Her eyes are sad. After a deep breath, she starts telling me about a feeling of being neglected at the hospital. A feeling of neither being invited into the care of her mother nor into the decisions made on treatment. She thinks it might be because she herself is a nurse. The staff might be scared of her, she thinks.

I just listen. I have a sense that she needs to tell me everything. I sense anger and powerlessness in her words while she tells me about being overlooked and even blamed for her wish to participate in the care of her mother. She tells me about frustrations of knowing how certain medicaments affect her mother—and about a feeling that no one listens or acknowledges her specific knowledge.

I am a bit alert . . . where does this conversation lead us?

I notice that her old mother has closed her eyes, as if she wants to withdraw.

After a while of just listening, the daughter calms down.

Everything becomes silent . . .

After a while, I quietly ask if she is ready to start all over again in a fellowship and joint effort with me. I also carefully mention that I think her mother is very ill and needs both her daughter and us as caregivers.

She leans back and heaves a sigh.

She seems empty for words and extremely tired.

Her eyes carry no anger anymore and she seems to open herself towards me—just by the way she is sitting in the chair—right there, in front of me.

QUESTIONS I CARE ABOUT

The above lived-experience description is an excerpt from a philosophical essay written by Sofia, a nurse who participated in a phenomenological action-research project on moments of beauty in nursing (Herholdt-Lomholdt, 2018, 2019). The aim of this former research was to enquire into moments of beauty to reach a deeper understanding of the nature of beauty in nurses' practice and nurse-patient relations. For half a year, Sofia, fourteen other nurses involved in the project, and I had philosophical conversations and essayistic writing processes centred on this and similar situations.[1] The above description is a small picture of a moment of beauty in Sofia's daily practice as a nurse.

The project—which was my doctoral thesis—was anchored in existential phenomenology (Max van Manen, 1990, 2014) and philosophical aesthetics (Jørgensen, 2010, 2012, 2014).

In this chapter, the purpose is to enquire further into a certain kind of experience within moments of beauty in nursing, which is also present in Sofia's description and essay, an experience in which something other than the nurse herself takes over and guides her way of being and acting. An experience in which, in short glimpses, these nurses give up on their own control and give themselves over to something other than themselves. And also a peculiar experience in which, in such glimpses of self-surrender, it feels as if there is a connection to something of everlasting value. In the thesis, I name such kinds of self-surrendering ways of being and acting as 'moved movements' (Herholdt-Lomholdt, 2018). In Sofia's description, it could be expressed by the way silence comes to existence, which I will return to in more depth throughout this chapter.

Approaching moments of beauty as moments where human beings and situations as such flourish, the main questions raised in this chapter are: How can we describe and understand such experiences of 'something other' taking over? How is it possible to comprehend that which is taking over? Moreover, are such non-decided ways of being and acting ethical? If so, how can we then comprehend such kinds of ethics? By following these leading questions, I hope to invite the reader into thoughtful considerations on how and where human flourishing can take place in professional work and relations.

MOMENTS OF BEAUTY IN NURSING: A PLACE FOR MOVED MOMENTS AND SELF-SURRENDER

From the beginning, I will try to avoid some possible misunderstandings concerning moments of beauty in nursing. As can be seen in Sofia's story, moments of beauty are not essentially pretty, harmonic or well-functioning moments. Most often, they start out being foggy and through which it is difficult to find a way. Often, moments of beauty arise in situations of enormous human loss, anxiety, and powerlessness. In the midst of that, when everything is imbued with darkness, glimpses of life and light sometimes find their own surprising way. This also means that moments of beauty are beyond human control. A nurse cannot decide to create moments of beauty. They merely happen to us. In that sense, a moment of beauty is a precious and enigmatic gift.

However, if the beauty in these moments is not just beautiful or enjoyable, then how can we then describe it?

Relying on the philosophic aesthetic work of Dorthe Jørgensen (Jørgensen, 2009, 2010, 2011, 2012, 2014, 2008) and experiences expressed through my doctoral thesis, I approach moments of beauty as a certain kind of *world-disclosive experience*, where we as persons (in this context, nurses) receive a glimpse of something of common and everlasting value. In the dissertation, I describe such world-disclosive experiences as moments where nurses get a sense of overwhelming meaningfulness, a sense arising suddenly and non-decided in the midst of the ordinary daily practice of nursing. Right there, within all the trivialities, something valuable and worth noticing becomes present.

Jørgensen describes such moments as a metaphysical experience, further developed with her concept of "a surplus of meaning"(Jørgensen, 2011 p. 5). A surplus of meaning is handed over to us in these moments, a surplus of meaning that exceeds the situation as such and goes beyond what human beings are capable of creating themselves. Metaphysics in this sense does not refer to an outer or upper world inaccessible to human beings. Instead, metaphysics refers to a mundane metaphysic based on the thoughts of Heidegger (1929) and, in a Nordic context, also stated by the philosopher and theologian K. E. Løgstrup (1995, 2012). Metaphysics is, in this sense, an exceeding dimension present in our ordinary life.

This also means that moments of beauty are more than a private or subjective experience. Moments of beauty exceed the subject–object dichotomy and are, as Jørgensen puts it, sudden and overwhelming experiences of a fullness of meaning given to us in small and sometimes even surprising glimpses, e.g., as glimpses of hope, laughter, joy, and love—but also of powerlessness, sorrow, and anxiety.[2]

One of the main findings in the thesis is that in moments of beauty in nursing, nurses seem to be and become embodied resonance, with a surplus of meaning arising within the situation. The glimpse of meaning, which is characteristic of moments of beauty, seems to have an effect on the way nurses move, talk, and act (see also Herholdt-Lomholdt, 2019). Is it a situation imbued with sorrow or anxiety, as it might have been in Sofia's case, nurses move slowly and quietly. Is it a situation filled with joy, nurses move differently and in another tempo. And in situations that have reached a deadlock, hitherto unknown ways of being, sometimes find their way through the body and voice of the nurse.

This might seem self-evident, but what I find so remarkable is that the nurses are not fully aware of their altered way of being present. Actually, it seems as if the nurses do not at all *decide* to move slowly and quietly in moments of sorrow and despair. It merely seems to happen to them! It really is as if something *other* takes over. As mentioned earlier, I name such kinds of non-decided and self-surrendering being *moved movements*.

The question now is how it is possible to further describe and understand this peculiar place in professional life, where nurses momentarily give themselves over to something 'other,' while at the same time giving up on being in full control or mastery? How is it possible to describe and comprehend that which moves them?

In the thesis, I briefly discuss these questions with the late writings of the French philosopher Maurice Merleau-Ponty and point to his concept of 'the heart of being' (Merleau-Ponty, 2000) as a mystery from which acts, movements and words can be inspired (Herholdt-Lomholdt, 2018, 2019). In the thesis, I end up taking a tiny step from a purely aesthetic approach to a more religious or theological questioning by asking: Who or what is it that moves or call forth such moved movements? Or, put differently, who or what is this 'other'? In Merleau-Ponty's own reflections on these complicated questions, religion or theology do not play a great role. Nevertheless, in his late writings on art, he starts using Egyptian mythology and even dares to use the word 'God' as a possible source, without ever going into any definitions of God (see, as an example, Merleau-Ponty, 2000, p. 61ff). Nevertheless, Merleau-Ponty never gets clear about ethics or metaphysics, and therefore his writings—also his late writings—are limited when it comes to shedding light on these nurses' experiences. In the following, therefore, I will follow the same questions, but now by turning towards other philosophical and theological landscapes.

ON THE BORDER BETWEEN A THEOLOGICAL AND A PHILOSOPHICAL AESTHETIC APPROACH

In what follows, I will place the questions on otherness, self-surrender, and ethics in moments of beauty in nursing between a philosophical aesthetic and a theological approach by taking a closer look at the notions of call, response and the voice of 'an other,' based on the writings of Jean-Louis Chrétien.[3] By doing so, I hope to deepen the understanding of a possible connection between moved movements and ethics, as such a connection might shed further light on a possible place for human flourishing in nursing as well as other health professions.[4,5]

Chrétien's work belongs to a tradition in France called the new 'radicalised phenomenology' (Davenport, 2004), a tradition described and critically discussed as a theological turn in French phenomenology in the 1990s (Janicaud et al., 2000). The theological turn was—and still is—criticised because of its focus on experiences of the divine and different kinds of passages to God, e.g., through prayer and praise (Courtine, 2000). Recognising the critique, I dare to go with Chrétien in his descriptions of human experiences of glimpses of a revelation from infinity and the presence of an 'other' within these experiences. Based on religious experiences of prayer and aesthetic experiences of beauty, Chrétien tries to unveil and present a phenomenology of a common human experience of being *given—and given over* to something, a 'something' that is hard—maybe even impossible—to describe in words (Chrétien, 2000, 2004). Inspired by Dorthe Jørgensen (Jørgensen, 2014), I approach such experiences as common human experiences, available for all kinds of people, religious as well as non-religious, thereby also available in the everyday life of nurses.

As a reader, you might have some reservations. You might ask whether it is necessary to bring in theology or religious interpretations. You might critically ask, do I have to be a believer to accept the premises of this chapter? To both questions, I would say 'no.'

As Jørgensen puts it, different interpretations are both possible and likely. Nevertheless, neglecting an approach towards the interface between theology and philosophical aesthetics might also be a neglect of something of possible value. As Jørgensen argues, in a world with an increasing search for something that can serve as reference points, it seems difficult to live a good life with a reference point towards nothing (Jørgensen, 2014, p. 613). While theology qualifies by offering a reference point of something or someone absolute although not necessarily expressible, philosophic aesthetics qualify by anchoring such reference points in our lived experiences of immanent transcendence.

By placing this chapter in the interface between theology and philosophical aesthetics, I am searching for words to describe a common human experience of being called or given over to something or something 'other.' And I am searching for an ethical reference point beyond human beings, without defining this 'beyond human beings' too narrowly or unequivocally.

Three main steps will guide the rest of the chapter. First, I will return to Sofia's lived experience description (Van Manen, 1990; 2014) with some phenomenological openings and questions. Secondly, these openings and questions will be explored through the lenses of Chrétien and discussed through the lens of the French philosopher Paul Ricoeur. Finally, a possible interconnection between moved movements, ethics, and human flourishing will be suggested.

SOPHIA AND MOVED MOVEMENTS

In the following, I will go deeper into Sofia's lived-experience description and essay as such. In the description at the beginning of this chapter, we get only some of Sofia's story and reflections. As her essay continues, she writes more about the context and surroundings. Sofia describes how she at first enters the old woman's room at the hospital with an energy differing strikingly from the atmosphere already in the room. Sofia writes about herself as a nurse who, earlier that day, started out trying to take the room and make it hers. She writes about a wish to bring sun, warmth, and happy feelings into the room.

Nevertheless, within the very first minute, while Sofia draws back some white and transparent curtains, she realises that something else is at stake in this room, something she describes as 'a coolness, darkness, something pale, enclosed, tired and tacit' (Sofia's essay, translated by the author). The atmosphere in the room is described as fundamentally different from Sofia's mood.

A remarkable point in Sofia's story and essay is that, intertwined in her sense of coolness, hesitation, and darkness, she suddenly *finds* herself being silent. She describes how she suddenly stops humming and trying to force sunshine into the room. She describes this change as *happening to her* non-willingly. In her continuing essay, she even describes a peculiar experience of *silence finding her,* as if silence has an existence on its own. Sofia writes:

> Silence comes towards us automatically . . . it is just coming—almost as an afterthought, placed to help us find our way . . . it is like silence itself speaks and walks ahead of me. (Sofia's essay, author's translation)

This remarkable sense of a silence placed to help Sofia and that walks ahead of her is also present in the quoted lived-experience description at the beginning. At first, Sofia describes how she intentionally expresses herself. She actively chooses to tell about her approach to the daughter as co-hospitalised, and decides to describe the different kinds of services she will offer.

However, throughout her description, silence seems to knock on the door. When Sofia realises that she is not even able to get up from the chair, she surrenders and silence takes over. I now wonder if silence really was as irresistible as it seemed in that moment? Does this silence really exceed Sofia's own will?

In Sofia's continuing essay, she reflects on the meaning of silence as she senses that, through this non-chosen silence, a precious gift is given to her and the daughter. Sofia also describes how this remarkable gift of silence brings her closer to the situation and the daughter. By bumping into a chair, not knowing what to do, something happens. When something or someone makes Sofia silent, when something or someone calls Sofia to stop her flow of words, the situation changes. When Sofia surrenders, a turning point emerges. From there, a new beginning starts to take form, obviously not guided by the will of Sofia or the daughter. A new beginning just happens to them while they briefly sit together in silence. From there, from a silence that Sofia did not create but strangely could not avoid stepping into, something slowly but surely changes. The daughter starts to entrust Sofia her story and Sofia receives it.

In what follows, I will not specifically reflect on the phenomenon of silence, although it is extremely interesting. What I want to reflect on is this amazing description of silence as a gift that Sofia could not refuse. I will reflect on the experience of something being given and at the same time being given over to the given. It is as if this 'something' is able to both call upon and change Sofia's way of being in a very concrete and embodied way. Sofia experiences becoming another nurse, twisted out of her spontaneous joyful and humming nurse-self, towards a silent and listening way of being present. Sofia momentarily becomes another version of herself.

SILENCE AS AN EMBODIED RESPONSE

I will start out by concentrating on Sofia's experience of finding herself being silent, placed within silence and given over to silence, which she does not decide to enhance by her own conscious will.

In nursing research, it is surely provocative to focus on ways of acting and being that are out of nurses' control. Through the last decade, concepts like clinical decision-making, clinical judgment, and other similar concepts have been raised to underline the importance of nurses who, conscious of and grounded in their professional knowledge, *choose* how to act and behave (see as an example Benner, Tanner, & Chesla, 1996; Gillespie & Peterson, 2009; Gray, 2001; Taylor, Dowding, & Johnson, 2017; Thompson m.fl., 2001).

Sofia's story gives a glimpse of a being that sneaks underneath or beyond the sphere of conscious choice. Sofia describes how she *finds* herself being silent and brought to a stand-still, and she writes about a peculiar experience of silence finding her. As a reader, I am intrigued by Sofia's descriptions of a silence and stoppage that enter her whole body non-willingly. She did not at first hear or sense something that she secondly decided to react to. Actually, she expresses it the other way round: silence finds her and she finds herself within silence. She finds her mouth shut and her body anchored to a chair. Silence seems to find her by entering her whole body. Her movements, which earlier were so busy, suddenly stop. Her words, trying to comfort the daughter, stop. The whole situation becomes silent, as an event. I think silence finds Sofia by presenting itself *through* her and by *surrounding* her. By making Sofia's body silent, silence seems to enhance her listening capability. It is as if silence presents itself with its own will, a will that in a short glimpse takes the lead.

CHÉTIEN AND THE RESPONSE

Based on Sofia's reflections and seen through the lens of Chrétien, it is possible to suggest that Sofia finds herself in a *response* (Chrétien, 2004). Reading Chrètien, I understand that his concept of a response carries three main characteristics:

1. At first, one could think a response is an intentional answer to something or someone, an answer formed by us as human beings. Nevertheless, this is not the case in Chrétien's work. A response is not the result of a decision, but something we find ourselves within. A response happens to us suddenly as an answer that flows through us. Chrétien describes the response as a 'springing into being' (Chrétien, 2004, p. 17), and this 'springing' is not intentional. It merely happens to us, like Sofia describes silence happening to her, a 'spring' that just comes forth.
2. According to Chrétien, such a non-willed response holds self-overcoming potential (Davenport, 2004, p. xii). The response makes us become more than what we are—or more fully what we are. Although we are present as fully ourselves in the response, we exceed ourselves as well. Chrétien writes it in a rather cryptic manner: 'The space of response is opened only by the difference between speaking of oneself and

speaking oneself' (Chrétien, 2004, p. 27). And later, with a reference to Heidegger, he writes: 'I myself speak, without speaking from myself' (Chrétien, 2004, p. 29). The point here is that something more—something other—than our usual selves comes to presence in the response, as 'an idea of myself that was before I was' (ibid., p. 24) and, by stepping into this idea, 'an irreparable and fugitive resonance' emerges (Chrétien, 2004, p. 83). In response, a 'larger self' or a more fully me self seems to arise and can, according to Chrétien, bring us in a renewed—although fugitive—resonance with the wholeness of the situation.

By reading Chrétien's rather cloudy texts on this issue, I sense some kind of resonance with Sofia's experience of being given over to a silent way of being. An experience of being and becoming a self, other than she used to be. An experience of this silent becoming, which she did not choose but opened herself to, which enabled a renewed and precious contact with the tired daughter.

3. Finally, according to Chrètien, a response is not just verbatim, but involves our whole body and soul, 'the whole flesh,' as Chrétien writes with a reference to Merleau-Ponty (Chrétien, 2004, p. 83). This means that Sofia's embodied silence, while finding herself bound to a chair, can be comprehended as an example of an embodied response.

The question now is, if the silence within and around Sofia is comprehended as an embodied and self-overcoming response, who or what is she responding to? In other words, who or what triggered the silence to flow through Sofia? Who or what is it that calls forth such self-overcoming responses?

SILENCE AS A RESPONSE TO A CALL

It seems obvious to connect Sofia's silence with the tired daughter. The daughter needed room for sharing her frustrations and thoughts, and Sofia responded by being a silent listener. In that sense, it is possible to describe Sofia's response as being to the daughter and an expression of Sofia's empathic capability.

Empathy is often, at least in nursing, understood as the ability to sense the 'private perceptual world' of the other, as Carl Rogers describes it (Rogers, 1962, 1975, p. 4). From such an approach, the trigger for silence is connected to the daughter and the situation of the mother and daughter. Silence is, in that sense, a response to a cry or call coming from the mother and her daughter. In spite of this, in the following, I will show that moved movements and the approach of Chrétien goes further and beyond empathy in Roger's sense.

As mentioned in the beginning of this chapter and with a reference to Jørgensen (2014, 2015), moved movements connect to something more than empathy. They relate to a sphere that exceeds ontic situations and human relations, although coming to presence within ontic situations and human relations. Moved movements are not solely triggered by the presence of other persons. They also rely on a sensitivity towards something 'more,' towards a surplus of meaning arising within the moment (Herholdt-Lomholdt, 2018). This surplus of meaning could, in Sofia's case, be silence as an ontological life phenomenon.

Chrétien's work goes one step further by introducing a *call* (Chrétien, 2004). Following Chrétien, it is possible to say that there is a call *behind* the silence. If silence is comprehended as a response, then silence is an answer. An answer to what? To a call, Chrètien would say.

How can we understand the kind of call that Chrètien writes about? The call is not from a voice we can hear, and it is not through words (Davenport, 2004). It's not a call from the daughter, the nurse herself, the mother or the phenomena of silence itself. Actually, the call leaves me short of words to describe it, because the call is on the one hand silent and, on the other hand, severe and present.

According to Chrétien, one of the main characteristics of beauty is that it carries a call that addresses the wholeness of our being. It's 'a call *for* someone and *to* someone' (Chrétien, 2004, p. 5). The call cries an appeal, which is irresistible and at the same time caring (Chrétien, 2004, p. 14). The call is like a clang or echo that sings silently everywhere and through everything—and this clang addresses us.

Moreover, when we are addressed by a call, it has connotations of something more than what is visible or audible. The call points to an exceeding metaphysical dimension. The call addresses us here and now and is in that sense concrete. At the same time, the call, according to Chrètien, carries a sound from eternity (Chrétien, 2004, p. 21).

Expressed by the words of Chrétien, 'Beauty therefore calls and recalls indeed by its very essence' (Chrétien, 2004, p. 14). By using the notion of a '*re-call,*' Chrétien points to the call as actually two calls: a primary or first call and a re-call. Behind and within the re-call is a *first call*, also described merely as an original call.

The first call is comprehended by Chrètien as a call from non-being into being. The first and original call called us—and everything—from non-existence into existence. The first call is a call to be at all.

Every re-call, as the call behind Sofia's silence, is also a call into existence (Chrétien, 2004, p. 17), a reverberation of the first call. The re-call is a call that draws man out of nothingness, calling human beings into existence (ibid., p. 22). Both calls are calls to become. The first call called us into existence.

The re-call is a 'recalling us to ourselves' (ibid., p. 10). In that sense, the re-call makes it possible for us to become more fully what we are.

When we are called, we are called 'from time immemorial,' says Chrétien (2004, p. 24). The call is in touch with something that exceeds the concrete situation, though still based on it. The call is more than a call from this certain situation and more than a call arising from this certain mother and daughter. Although present in this situation, the call connects to something larger than it.

However, we do not directly hear the first call or the re-call. In that sense, the call and recall are silent. What we sense is a response flowing through us. According to Chrètien, we have no access to the call as such, and therefore, it is not possible for us to either express, point to or give any intentional or conscious answers to the call. Nevertheless, through the response that flows through us, we realise that we have been addressed by a call which we are not able to utter.

Chrétien's description of the interconnection between a call and a response can shed light on Sofia's almost mysterious description of being wrapped up in silence in a non-decided way. The silence coming to presence through Sofia's altered voice and body is, in Chrétien's sense, a response to a re-call to which Sofia has access only through her embodied response. Sofia does not hear the call; neither does she intentionally form an answer. Sofia rather finds herself in response to a call of which she does not consciously know, answering it by being silent.

WHO OR WHAT IS CALLING?: AN ECHO FROM ETERNITY

The question now is, who or what is calling within such experiences of silently being called?

According to Chrétien, the call manifests and points towards an origin 'over itself' (Chrétien, 2004, p. 37). Experiences of being called point towards a presence of something original and maybe even absolute. In Chrétien's sense, the call carries an echo from the morning the world was created. As a believer, he points to the presence of a creative power in the first call, the call from non-being into being. Chrétien also points to this power as one that resonates in every re-call in the world. In that sense, the call is somehow both majestic and silent, powerful and at the same time non-audible.

Without being too specific in definitions of such creative power, Chrètien names this presence as an echo from eternity that sings from and to eternity through a call and into our human response. In that sense, the silence flowing through Sofia is a situated, very concrete and embodied way of being present in a hospital room. At the same time, the silence could be connected to a clang or echo that has whispered from eternity.

Ethics is, in Chretien's approach, connected to this call from eternity. Ethics are in that sense not something human beings solely create, construct or decide. Ethics are connected to something or someone eternal, a presence beyond human beings, to which all human beings have access. In other texts, he describes this echo from eternity and the creative power as an endless love. This means that although the call and response come to presence in-between a nurse and a tired daughter on an ordinary day and at an ordinary hospital ward, it is not just them being present. Something more, described as love, eternity, and care, comes to presence as well, and this 'more' enters the room through Sofia's embodied response. Sofia's silence can in that sense be comprehended as a silence carried by love and care.

This means that in the work of Chrètien, the structure of a call and response points to an ethical dimension that exceeds the situation as such, a dimension that exceeds every situation and goes on forever. The embodied and very concrete response can in that sense be comprehended as the gate wherein something infinite, a 'spirit,' makes itself present in a finite world. Chrétien writes:

> The original call, the call that delivers us and sends us into the world, can only be perceived in our unavoidably belated response, through our own altered voice. . . . This voice, our own, the human voice where we listen forever to what beckons to us, is the very place where the spirit erupts into the world. In the timbre of the voice, spirit manifests itself the only way that is possible for it, which is body and soul. It gives itself by uttering itself. (Chrétien, 2004, p. 44)

The spirit Chrétien writes about in the above citation is what has earlier in this chapter been described as a creative power, an echo from eternity and an endless love. He also names this power 'God'; in other texts, he cautiously and maybe more open for secular people describes this presence as a voice of an 'Other'.[6] Chrétien thereby positions the call and response in relation to someone or something eternal and 'Other' than both human and culture. Chrétien anchors ethics to this Otherness. Chrétien's position is, in that sense, religious, based on a Catholic approach and theology, although in quite an open manner.

This means that in the work of Chrétien, the voice of the Other is not solely an injunction coming from other human beings. In his optic, the voice of the Other places us in an order superior to ourselves and other human beings as such. In the experience of call and response, we are not just affected by a dialogue with ourselves, nor just by a dialogue with other human beings. In the call, we are also addressed by something infinite and even absolute. The presence of this Other is, according to Chrétien, crucial as 'the condition of my humanity' (Chrétien, 2004, p. 81).

According to Chrétien, the voice of the radical Other does not dictate the actions of human beings, but calls us again and again to translate the absolute, love and care, into a changeable world. According to Chrétien, we do not hear the first call, nor do we have direct access to the absolute. What we hear or sense is our translation taking form as a response, and in this translation we get a sense of something that 'we are not the sources of,' as Chrétien puts it (Chrétien, 2004, p. 44). As Chretien thoughtfully writes, the most empirical aspect of the call, meaning the experience of being addressed and given over to something is also the most transcendent aspect (Chrétien, 2004, p. 81).

WHO OR WHAT IS CALLING US TO RESPOND? A CALL FROM AN OTHER

In French phenomenology, the theological turn in Chrétien's work is discussed and criticised, among others, by Paul Ricoeur (2000). Ricoeur, who was himself a believer, does acknowledge that human beings have feelings of meeting something absolute (e.g., as a sense of dependence, belonging or utter confidence in spite of suffering). Ricoeur also acknowledges that such feelings can point towards the existence of an origin different from humanity and culture, one over human beings and their experience.

Nevertheless, Ricoeur criticises the way theology, on phenomenological grounds, uses such experiences to describe or point towards an origin to which we have no direct access and therefore can give words only through several layers of cultural, historic and linguistic interpretations (Ricoeur, 2000). In that sense, Ricoeur critiques the way Chrétien uses the experiences of beauty and prayer to point towards an existence that no one can see or sense directly. Ricoeur writes:

> My presupposition does not say that nothing can be taken as religious 'experience'—be it a feeling of 'absolute dependence,' a response to a will that precedes me, an 'ultimate concern' at the horizon of all my decisions, or 'an unconditional confidence' that hopes in spite of . . . everything. These are some of the synonyms of what has been called faith, those at least that are most familiar and closest to me. So understood, faith is certainly not an act that can be reduced to any act of speaking or any piece of writing. . . . But the presupposition of listening to Christian preaching is not that everything is language; it is rather that it is always within language that religious experience is articulated, that one hears it in a cognitive, practical or emotional sense. . . . In one sense, therefore, text does precede life. I can name God in my faith because the texts preached to me have already named God. (Ricoeur, 1995, p. 218)

Although acknowledging that there might be a presence of something or someone Other, which is worth our faith, Ricoeur is more careful when it comes to pointing towards it than Chrétien. I can only name it because our culture and history already have named it, Ricoeur says Ricoeur is in that way much more careful when it comes to giving words to the sense of absoluteness.

At the same time, Ricoeur also describes ethics as relying on 'an other,' and he puts forth the presence of otherness as an important and common human experience (Ricoeur, 1992). The question, then, is who or what is this 'other' calling upon us, in Ricoeur's sense? And how is this kind of otherness connected to ethics?

In the book *Oneself as Another*, Ricoeur introduces his thoughts of ethics as "aiming at the 'good life' with and for others, in just institutions" (1992, p. 172). Ricoeur unfolds the aspects of ethics as superior to morals and norms by discussing the notion of a 'good life,' the relation with and for others and his thoughts of just institutions.

The notion of a good life is, in Ricoeur's sense, connected to a reflexivity that moves between our aim of a good life on the one hand and our particular choices on the other. Nevertheless, this reflexivity cannot stand alone. The good life is not just connected with me. It must be seen in the light of the next part of the sentence: a good life *with and for others.*

By writing that, Ricoeur points to ethics as anchored in relation to others. The other is, in Ricoeur's sense, another self, meaning another human being. The other plays a mediating role in-between the ability to make reflexive judgments and the actual act. Ethics are, in Ricoeur's sense, based in solicitude and mutuality and anchored in the presence of another human being and in human beings as such. In his book *Figuring the Sacred* (Ricoeur, 1995), Ricoeur argues that the Golden Rule, as it is formulated in different biblical texts, must be the 'supreme principle of morality' (Ricoeur, 1995 p. 293). In that sense, ethics are based on intersubjectivity. Ethics are in Ricoeur's sense relational. Ethics come to presence in interactions with others. The other can be a 'victim of my action as much as its adversary' (Ricoeur, 1995, p. 294).

According to Ricoeur, reflexivity without solicitude and mutuality carries a risk of being self-sufficient and enclosed. The resources of goodness 'spring forth only from a being who does not detest itself to the point of being unable to hear the injunction coming from the other' (Ricoeur, 1992, p. 189). Ethical goodness and an ethical sense can, in the light of Ricoeur, only be judged by the way an act is done out of regards for others (p. 189). Seen through the lens of Ricoeur, ethics rely on a reflexive solicitude with and for other human beings aiming at a 'good life'—not just for me, but for all of us. Ethics esteem 'the other as oneself' and 'oneself as another' (Ricoeur, 1992, p. 194). In Sofia's case, there are reasons to believe that Ricoeur would describe 'the other' as both the daughter, her mom and as suffering human beings as such. In the texts I refer to, Ricoeur does not use the word call, but instead 'injunction.' Ethics is, in Ricoeur's sense, connected to an injunction coming from another self and a reflexive way of answering it.

SOPHIA, ETHICS, AND HUMAN FLOURISHING

Sofia's lived-experience description and essay, describing a peculiar experience of being disrupted by silence while being busy doing other things, is filled with wonder. Sofia herself describes the situation as an ethical event. She experienced that the silence flowing through her was a gift of ethical value. Something more was given with this silence: a connection, a trust, a new beginning . . .

Following the words of Chrétien and Ricoeur, it is possible to shed different sorts of light on Sofia's experience.

On the one hand, it is possible to say that being a good nurse in this specific situation relies on the way silence becomes present *through* Sofia. Sofia experiences a call through her own response. In this call, there might be a presence of something infinite, maybe a creative power or infinite love that exceeds Sofia, the culture of the hospital ward—even her relation to the daughter. Through Sofia's response, by being silent and a silent listener, she might be placed in an order that exceeds what she could ever have created herself. Ethics can, in this sense, be understood as a response to a call raised by some kind of eternal love. Ethics is in this sense pre-cultural given by a spirit to which we have no direct access, and at the same time ethics enter our world through a non-conscious translation of the infinite into a finite response.

On the other hand, the voice of the other is not necessarily a divine word, but also an injunction raised through the relation between the daughter, the mother and Sofia. The other would, in Ricoeur's sense, be the daughter, her mom and mankind as such, and Sofia's act of silence could be comprehended as a reflexive act done concerning the daughter, an act and response based on solicitude with another self. Ethics is, in this sense, a response to a call raised primarily around another human being.

Both comprehensions acknowledge and recognise Sofia's experience of something other taking the lead in the situation. Both comprehensions put forth that the presence of otherness is of affectional meaning when it comes to ethics. In that sense, both interpretations point towards a common human experience of being called by and towards the good.

The question is, do these different interpretations make any difference?

Chrétien's ethics go beyond human and cultural values and places our sense of the good in a pre-human and pre-cultural call. Although not denying the possible presence of the divine, Ricoeur's ethics are merely placed in-between human beings and within history, culture and solicitude. Does it make any difference whether we anchor ethics in a divine, loving and absolute voice of the Other or whether we stay on our earthly ground, so to speak, and primarily understand ethics as anchored in a solicitude with and a summons coming from other human beings? Put in other words, is a theological or religious interpretation necessary?

In the following, I will briefly discuss this issue on two levels, first on the level of Sofia's experience and second on a merely philosophical and theological level, by referring to the Danish philosopher, Løgstrup.

Looking upon Sofia's experience, it is possible to comprehend her response on both levels. The silence coming towards her can both be comprehended as a reflexive act driven by compassion (a word used by Ricoeur as well) and a non-intentional response that flows through her, driven by some kind of everlasting, absolute goodness or love. Both interpretations seem plausible based on Sofia's experience.

Sofia might act in continuity with the golden rule. Her silence might be doing to the daughter as she would have the daughter to do to her. At the same time, it seems possible to understand the ethics of the situation as more than solely relational and reflexive ethics in Ricoeur's sense. Something 'more' than the daughter and the mother was present in the situation, and this 'more' did not present itself to Sofia's conscious or reflective self.

Through discussions and philosophical conversations, both Sofia and the other nurses participating in the research expressed a feeling of being connected to something of everlasting value in moments of beauty, a sense of suddenly being in close interrelatedness with something 'more,' which was of life-threatening importance to hear and react to (see also Herholdt-Lomholdt, 2018), a sense of goodness which they did not and could not create through reflexivity and solicitude. Such experiences were described as exceeding. Through our dialogues, some participating nurses even expressed a need to thank something or someone for letting them be a part of such moments. These nurses did not express pride for being or doing good in moments of beauty. Often, as in Sofia's case, they actually did not act by themselves, and they expressed deep gratitude (for other examples of such senses of gratitude and its connection to 'the holy,' see also Martinsen [2018]).

In that sense, and relying on the words of Chrétien, it is possible to say that Sofia becomes truly herself by lending her voice and body to a response to a call, which could involve the voice of a radical Other. Nevertheless, this 'Other' presents itself only *within* Sofia's altered voice and body. It whispers in silence and is a mystery. Surely, such an approach is a question of firm belief.

IS A THEOLOGICAL OR RELIGIOUS INTERPRETATION OF A CALL NECESSARY?

In the work of the Danish philosopher and theologian Løgstrup, the question of the necessity of religious interpretations is also raised. He writes about the so-called sovereign life utterances (e.g., trust), that their presence makes religious interpretations obvious but not necessary (Løgstrup, 1995, p. 211). What Løgstrup points to here is that the presence of trust, for example, is a possible experience for everyone. Trust does not need any theological wrapping to be present in our lives. Trust is present and recognisable for everyone as a common human experience. Løgstrup then raises a question like the one raised here: What do we lose if we lay aside religious interpretations?

And he answers thoughtfully: We would lose nothing!

At first glance, this statement seems to compromise religious interpretations. It does not make any difference at an ethical level whether we consider ethics as based in something absolute (an Other in Chrétien's sense) or solely in solicitude with and for other human beings (an other in Ricoeur's sense). But actually this is not what Løgstrup says.

On the question, why we lose nothing by neglecting religious interpretations, his answer is surprising. According to Løgstrup, we lose nothing because the active power within the sovereign life utterances is not dependent on our religious interpretations (Løgstrup, 1995, p. 215). In other words, what is given to us is given no matter. It's not our belief that calls the sovereign life utterances to life, just as it's not we who call the call into existence in the work of Chrètien. This means that the reason we will lose nothing is not because religious interpretations are false or unimportant, but because its sovereignty exceeds our firm beliefs. In Løgstrup's sense, goodness and love will call us and we will respond to it, even if we are not believers. Or, as Løgstrup writes, 'The created life takes its course, irrespective of whether the individual believes or does not believe that it is created' (Løgstrup, 1995, p. 215, author's translation into English).

Of course, Løgstrup's answer to these questions can be perceived as rather arrogant and self confirming. I don't think this is the case. I think the case here is that it really is a question of firm belief whether we approach the call as a presence of an other in Ricoeur's sense or an Other in Chrétien's sense. But they both point to an important common human experience of being called and giving oneself over to something or someone other/Other. And they both point to a close interrelatedness between ethics and the experience of letting go of oneself—giving ourselves momentarily in service to this otherness.

Nevertheless, I will ask again: is Løgstrup right? Do we really lose nothing by setting aside the possibility of the presence of an Other in the call?

Going back to Sofia and the other nurses' descriptions and reflections, I would say: Yes, we might lose one thing by neglecting the possibility of a theological wrapping. We might lose a place where pride over human holdings can be replaced by a comprehensive gratitude. We might lose someone or somewhere to thank.

Despite that, it seems of importance, on the basis of both Chrétien's and Ricoeur's interpretations, to point to human flourishing in nursing as relying on much more than professional knowledge, good planning or relational capabilities. At its foundation, human flourishing relies on letting go of oneself and being open towards the presence of something or someone other. This other could either be other human beings but may also be the radical Other, as an echo from eternity or an endless love, an openness towards goodness, care, and love that is not solely linked to us but to that which is coming towards us.

The last question will now be how nurses and healthcare professionals can open themselves to, or grasp the call or injunction coming from, such voices external to themselves.

IF THE CALL IS SILENT, THEN HOW IS IT POSSIBLE TO LISTEN TO IT?

In the following, I will mainly turn to the work of Chrètien to discuss which attitudes or kinds of presence can enhance the possibility of hearing or responding to a call. As mentioned earlier, the call is not present as a voice like the voices we normally use when we speak. The voice of the call is in that sense silent. Instead, we can see—or sense—the call through our response, and our senses 'see truly only by listening' (Chrétien, 2004, p. 35). The question then is, how can we characterise such a kind of listening?

To hear the call behind our response means to listen further and elsewhere, to listen in a vast manner. It is a listening that 'exceeds by far the sense of hearing. Everything in us listens, because everything in the world and of the world speaks' (Chrétien, 2004, p. 14). Listening exceeds the hearing sense, and it means listening with and towards a wholeness.

In Sofia's case, this listening capability seems to be anchored in her whole body. Her legs, anchored to the chair, listens. Her mouth, suddenly silent, listens. Her feelings, sensing the atmosphere in the room, listen.

Chrétien develops the notion of a 'listening eye' to describe the listening capability (Chrétien, 2004, p. 33 ff). By using the notion of a listening eye, Chrétien wants to mark how every sense merges into one another while listening to an exceeding call from elsewhere. In Chrétien's sense, the 'listening eye' is neither connected to a conscious awareness nor a reflective attitude; it's not even connected to the eyes. It is merely understood as a listening arising from everywhere and directed towards everything, while being submerged within this very concrete moment.

At the same time, Chrétien points towards a paradox. By describing the listening eye, a possible misunderstanding lies near. The misunderstanding is that the call relies on a listening eye. But that is not the case. The call in itself is not dependent on any human listening capability. It is not we who call the call into existence. The call is always there—arising from every corner of our lives. The call is not preceded by any special kind of receptivity. Instead, our ability to hear the call relies on the fact that, as human beings, we always already carry the capability to listen. Chrétien writes:

> In other words, the call does not appeal to a pre-existing possibility in us of listening to it, as though it was inscribed in us in hollow, inversely and already called by us, as though we were the ones calling the call. It always brings itself its own possibility, which is to say the listener. (Chrétien, 2004, p. 22)

The paradox is that nurses—and healthcare personnel as such—ought to listen with all their senses, meaning their whole body and soul, to hear the call and respond to it. However, when they find themselves responding to a call, they realise that they are always already called. They realise that it is the call making them capable of listening and responding.

These reflections lead to the conclusion that no one can call the call. The call is always and already there. On the other hand, it is a possibility to resist having listening eyes—and thereby resist a response coming through. With a reference to the fourth-century philosopher Augustin, Chrétien recommends that we perform movements of withdrawal from the noise of the world and also calm down our own endless mumbling (Chrétien, 2004, p. 67). By doing so, he suggests that there might be a chance for the voice of the Other as well as the other to reach us and let us spring into being in ethical ways. Human flourishing, then, is characterised by moments in which a fugitive but valuable resonance with the situation, with the other and maybe even with some kind of everlasting love arises *through* us.

LETTING SPACES FOR ETHICAL RESPONSES IN HUMAN PROFESSIONS EMERGE: CLOSING REMARKS

This chapter points towards human flourishing as dependent on responsive spaces in healthcare professions and in human life as such: spaces in hospitals, kindergartens, and schools, where rules, regulations, guidelines, and other kinds of noises from the world can stand aside for ethical responses to flow through us; spaces that allow and enhance one to let go of oneself and let a voice from elsewhere reach us.

Human flourishing seems to rely on spaces where we let voices of otherness turn us as professionals to ourselves, by calling us to step into an ethical order that exceeds ourselves. Human flourishing seems to rely on spaces that make it possible to translate 'the origin' (Chrétien, 2004, p. 72) as well as solicitude with others (Ricoeur, 1992) into our modern world.

In that sense, human flourishing relies on responsive spaces, where professionals are allowed—or even encouraged—to spring into being, called by a word they cannot utter. In some ways, it places professionals in a paradoxical situation. On the one hand, we as humans do not call the call. On the other hand, we can fill our life, professions and selves with so much noise that we make it difficult for the voice of the other as well as the Other to reach us. As the call and response structure, with its exceeding dimensions, seems to make human growth and flourishing possible, it is also worth thinking whether the other way round is possible: can we become a 'smaller self' if we, or the organisations we are a part of, resist or hinder such responses to flow through us (Martinsen, 2020)?

In the future, it will be of main importance to question how institutions like hospitals and schools can enhance professionals who momentarily give themselves over to something other than themselves, to a call that they cannot directly define. How is it possible to enhance open and responsive spaces on two levels, the institutional level and the continuing formation of the professionals? This is a burning question and at the same time surely needed to let human life flourish in moments of joy as well as in moments of sorrow, anxiety, and despair.

ACKNOWLEDGMENTS

I want to thank the three editors of this book as well as professor Kari Martinsen for insightful readings and dialogues on the issues of this chapter.

NOTES

1. The form of these dialogues was inspired by Hansen's philosophical work on wonder and wonder-labs (see Hansen, 2008, 2012, 2015a, 2015b, 2017; Hansen & Sorrel Dinkins, 2016).

2. The surplus of meaning has a connection with, but is not identical to, feelings. The surplus of meaning is merely linked to the way the Danish professor of nursing, Charlotte Delmar, writes about ethical and existential life phenomena in nursing. Delmar differentiates both ethical and existential life phenomena from feelings. Whereas feelings allow us to understand other people and ourselves and give us access to life phenomena, life phenomena are understood as basic conditions for existence coming towards us. Life phenomena are, in Delmar's approach, given to us (Delmar, 2006).

3. Jørgensen also describes a 'calling' within the beauty-experience and briefly refers in this sense to the work of Chrétien (Jørgensen, 2014).

4. The 'call' in nursing has earlier been described by the Norwegian professor Kari Martinsen from a historic perspective and also inspired by Løgstrup (Martinsen, 2010). Martinsen's descriptions of a call is, in her earlier writings, primarily associated with a relational ethics based on Løgstrup's ethical demand (Løgstrup, 2012). The call is, in that optic, from the patient and a call to take care of the patient. In the following, the call is not solely linked to the other as other persons (e.g., the patient), but will also be described as a call coming from beyond the other and connected to a metaphysical surplus of meaning.

5. Scandinavian readers might ask why I turn to Chrètien when the Danish philosopher and theologian K.E. Løgstrup so clearly describes the phenomena of sovereign life utterances as given to human beings with life itself and as a foundation for ethical ways of being and becoming (Løgstrup, 2012). It is true that Løgstrup in many ways can shed light on a possible interconnection between moved movements and ethics, if we approach his concept of the sovereign life utterances as a kind of mediator between a pre-cultural and given ethics and moved movements, as movements guided by some kind of otherness. But in Løgstrup's work (Løgstrup, 1995), he operates with a separation of sensing and understanding, which I, from a position in philosophical aesthetics, do not rely on. In Løgstrup's work, human beings sense something and, based in those senses, they thoughtfully *form* an answer. Of course, this will be at stake very often. But from a philosophical aesthetic point of view, based on texts by Jørgensen and Baumgarten (Baumgarten, 1968; Jørgensen, 2014), moments of beauty are characterised by glimpses, where the distance between sensing and understanding is dissolved. The kind of understanding which comes to presence within these moments is of a different kind than a merely logical and cognitive recognition, and also different from any kind of conscious understanding. Baumgarten called it a 'sensitive recognition' and described with this concept another and aesthetic kind of understanding based on sensitivity with words as suspicions, clues, and feelings. The experience of moved movements, expressed through my dissertation, seems to be best expressed by Baumgarten's notion of sensitive recognition as a place where movements, senses, and understandings are totally intertwined without any internal distance.

6. According to Janicaud, French phenomenological theology often expresses the difference between 'the other' as culture and other human beings and 'the Other' as an exceeding and/or divine voice, by a difference in the use of a capital letter (Janicaud, 2000). In Chrétien's book on the call and response, he does not use capital letters, but very explicitly breaks with an understanding of 'the other' as solely other human

beings or culture. In the following parts of the chapter, I will use this difference in the use of capital letter to clarify when the other refers to culture and other human beings and when the Other refers to a more or less diffuse divinity.

REFERENCES

Baumgarten, A. G. (1968). Filosofiske betragtninger over digtet (P. A. Brandt & S. [translator] Kjørup [eds.]). Forlaget Arena.

Benner, P., Tanner, C. A., & Chesla, C. A. (1996). Expertice in Nursing Practice. Caring, Clinical Judgment, and Ethics. Springer Publishing Company.

Chrétien, J.-L. (2000). The wounded word: The Phenomenology of Prayer. In P. Janicaud, D., Courtine, J.F., Chrétien, J.L., Henry, M., Marion, J.L., Ricoeur (Ed.), Phenomenology and the "theological turn." The French Debate. (pp. 147–75). Fordham University Press.

Chrétien, J.-L. (2004). The Call and the Responce (Translated). Fordham University Press.

Courtine, J. F. (2000). Introduction: Phenomenology and Hermeneutics of Religion. In Phenomenology and the "theological turn." The French Debate. (pp. 121–26). Fordham University Press.

Davenport, A. A. (2004). Translator's Preface. In The Call and the Response (pp. vii–xxix). Fordham University Press.

Delmar, C. (2006). The phenomenology of life phenomena—in a nursing context. Nursing Philosophy, 7, 235–46.

Gillespie, M., & Paterson, B. L. (2009). Helping Novice Nurses Make Effective Clinical decision: The Situated Clinical Decision-Making Framework. Nursing Education Perspectives, 30(3), 164–70.

Gray, J. A. M. (2001). Evidence-based Healthcare (2nd ed.). Churcill Livingstone.

Hansen, F. T. (2008). At stå i det åbne. Dannelse gennem filosofisk undren og nærvær. Hans Reitzels Forlag.

Hansen, F. T. (2012). One step further: The dance between Poetic dwelling and Socratic wonder in Phenomenological Research. Indo-Pacific Journal of Phenomenology, 12, 1–20.

Hansen, F. T. (2015a). Når undringen leder til en fyldt stilhed, der er værd at tænke ud fra: Relevansen af "det Sokratiske" i humanvidenskab, højere uddannelse og professionsudvikling. Logos, 3(10), 7–14.

Hansen, F. T. (2015b). The Call and Practices of Wonder. How to evoke a Socratic Community of Wonder in Professional Settings. In M. N. Weiss (ed.), The Socratic Handbook. Dialogue Methods for Philosophical Practice. (pp. 217–44). LIT Verlag.

Hansen, F. T. (2017). Sokratisk og fænomenologisk orienteret aktionsforskning. In H. Alrø & F. T. Hansen (eds.), Dialogisk aktionsforskning i et praksisnært perspektiv (pp. 93–143). Aalborg Unviersitetsforlag.

Hansen, F. T., & Sorrel Dinkins, C. (2016). Socratic Wonder as a Way to Aletheia in Qualitative Research and Action Research. HASER. Revista Internacional de Filosofía Aplicada, 7, 51–88.

Heidegger, M. (1929). What is metaphysics. Oversat til engelsk af Miles Groth.
Herholdt-Lomholdt, Sine Maria. (2019). Invisible but sensible aesthetic aspects of excellence in nursing. Nursing Philosophy, 20(2). https://doi.org/10.1111/nup.12238.
Herholdt-Lomholdt, Sine Maria. (2018). Skønne øjeblikke i sygepleje—en kilde til innovation? En fænomenologisk og dialogisk aktionsforskningsundersøgelse af skønne øjeblikkes natur og mulige forbindelser til en sygeplejefaglig udviklings- og innovationspraksis. Aalborg University.
Janicaud, D. (2000). Contours of the turn. In Phenomenology and the "theological turn." The French Debate. (pp. 16–35). Fordham University Press.
Jørgensen, D. (2009). Why do we need philosphical aesthetics. Nordisk Tidsskrift for K, 17–34. https://doi.org/10.112/1.421275.
Jørgensen, D. (2010). The experience of immanent transcendence. Nordisk Tidsskrift for Kunst Og Kristendom, 11, 35–52. https://doi.org/10.112/1.421275.
Jørgensen, D. (2011). Verdenspoesi: Malerier og tankebilleder. Kvindemuseet Århus.
Jørgensen, D. (2012). Fornemmelsens filosofi: Æstetik, fænomenologi og erfarings-metafysik. In U. Thøgersen & B. Troelsen (eds.), Filosofi og kunst. (pp. 33–47). Aalborg Universitetsforlag.
Jørgensen, D. (2014). Den skønne tænkning. Veje til erfaringsmetafysik religionsfilosofisk undmøntet. Aarhus Universitetsforlag.
Jørgensen, D. (2015). Experiencem Metaphysics, and Immanent Transcendence. In D. Jørgensen, G. Chiurazzi, & S. Tinning (Eds.), Truth and Experience (pp. 11–30). Cambridge Scholars Publishing.
Jørgensen, D. (2008). Aesthetic thinking as a common humanist concern. Paper Presentation. The Symposium: "The Humanities in a New Era: Surviving or Setting the Agenda?" 1–5.
Løgstrup, K. E. (1995). Skabelse og tilintetgørelse. Religionsfilosofiske betragtninger. (2. udgave). Gyldendal.
Løgstrup, K. E. (2012). Den etiske fordring (4. udgave). Forlaget Klim.
Martinsen, K. (2010). Øjet og kaldet (2.). Munksgaard.
Martinsen, K. (2018). Bevegelig Berørt. Fagbokforlaget.
Martinsen, K. (2020). Readings of the call and response. E-mail correspondence.
Merleau-ponty, M. (2000). Artes. Øyet og ånden (T. by: M. B. Tin (ed.)). Pax Forlag A/S.
Ricoeur, P. (1992). Oneself as Another (K. [translator] Blamaey [ed.]). The University of Chicago Press.
Ricoeur, P. (1995). Figuring the Sacred. Religion, Narrative and Imagination. Fortress Press.
Ricoeur, P. (2000). Experience and Language in Religious Discourse. In Phenomenology and the "theological turn." The French Debate. (pp. 127–46). Fordham Univresity Press.
Rogers, C. (1962). The interpersonal Relationship: The Core of Guidance. Harvard Educational Review, 34(4), 416–29.
Rogers, C. R. (1975). Empathic: An Unappreciated Way of Being. The Counseling Psychologist, 5(2), 2–10. https://doi.org/10.1177/001100007500500202.

Taylor, P., Dowding, D., & Johnson, M. (2017). Clinical decision making in the recognition of dying: A qualitative interview study. BMC Palliative Care, 16(1). https://doi.org/10.1186/s12904-016–0179–3.

Thompson, C., McCaughan, D., Cullum, N., Sheldon, T. A., Mulhall, A., & Thompson, D. R. (2001). Research information in nurses' clinical decision-making: What is useful? Journal of Advanced Nursing, 36(3), 376–88. https://doi.org/10.1046/j.1365–2648.2001.01985.x.

van Manen, Max. (1990). Researching lived experience. Researching Lived Experience, 35–51.

van Manen, Max. (1990). Researching lived experience: Human science for an action sensitive pedagogy. SUNY Series in the Philosophy of Education, 8, 202. https://doi.org/10.1017/CBO9781107415324.004.

van Manen, Max. (2014). Phenomenology of practice. Meaning-giving methods in phenomenological research and writing. Left Coast Press.

Chapter 7

To Wonder about Something and to Be in Wonder

Two Different Approaches Explored by Applying Martin Buber's Philosophy of Dialogue

Aslaug Kristiansen

The Swedish award-winning novelist Ulf Stark (1944–2017) has written a wonderful children's book called *When Dad Showed Me the Universe* (2016). It is a delightful picture book illustrated by Eva Eriksson. The book tells the story about a father who wishes to show his little son the wonder and majesty of the universe on a star-studded night. The book starts at home as they prepare for the journey, and we follow father and son as they walk hand in hand through the town before they enter a meadow where the lights from the town no longer erode the light from the stars. The father lifts up his son and points out and names the stars in the sky. "You are supposed to look up," the father says, but while the father is looking up, the son explores the ground. He discovers the universe in a snail creeping over a stone, a blade of grass swaying in the wind, and the father's reflection in a tiny pond. There is more to the book, but I will not reveal its ending here. One could say that the father and son both discover the universe and are touched by it, but their presence and perspectives are different, and the state of wondering is not quite a shared experience. The son is fascinated by all the things he sees in front of him. The father has a goal for the walk; his gaze is directed upward toward the sky, where the stars are sparkling.

The book is beautifully written, with a warm sense of humour, and is worth reading. But as an educator, I wish to further explore some of the more philosophical and educational dimensions that the book embraces. We learn of a father who is keen to educate his son about the immensity of the universe. His son, however, has become tired and does not seem very interested. Has the journey become too long, or could it be the father's educational approach—the pointing and naming of the stars—that has caused the son to lose interest? In many ways, the father's role matches that of many educators. Educators often have expectations, a plan, a goal to fulfil, and a wish to share something they find exciting and worthwhile. When the students ask questions along the route, however, the teacher can sometimes be so focused on the goal that he or she is not able to perceive mysteries and to tune in to aspects along the way.

Metaphorically speaking, in today's school, much emphasis is placed on "gazing towards the goal," as well as on what kind of knowledge the student should be provided with at the end of the learning cycle. In the everyday life of schooling, the teacher develops robust and effective teaching methods to achieve the goal, and she or he is held accountable for the result and the quality of the learning process. To define a purpose and to suggest various teaching methods to achieve it is an approach similar to an instrumental and rational thinking process (Kristiansen, 2015). According to *Stanford Encyclopedia of Philosophy*, *instrumentalism* and *rationalization* mean, based on Weber's statements, a historical drive towards a world in which "one can, in principle, master all things by calculation." The relationship between human beings and nature is a subject-object relationship in which knowledge is considered an instrument for human control and mastery over nature (Gustavsson, 2001). Through the years in the field of education, there have been different interpretations of instrumental thinking. In today's situation, the connection to economic growth is made more explicit. The children should learn the necessary skills in crucial areas to become capable of entering a global job market and be able to live in a knowledge-driven economy (White paper Culture of learning [2003–2004]). Today, instrumentalism is present in almost all areas of human life. People are living in what Ilan Guur-Ze'ev (2005) describes as "a multicultural world governed by instrumental rationality and global capitalism" (Guur-Ze'ev, 2005, p. 21).

However, in the school today, there are still pockets or breathing spaces where a state of wonder can suddenly occur and could disturb the educational order. The following story, written by Mats Granath (1988), provides a beautiful example of this.

WHEN A DEAD MOUSE GETS IN THE WAY OF A GOOD PLAN

Mats Granath (1988) tells a story that has become a classic in the Nordic preschool teacher education. He once took a group of children for a walk in the forest with the intention of teaching them about autumn. The children were to pick leaves and learn about trees before going inside to draw, make prints and paint. But suddenly there is a barrier that would upset any teacher's plans; the path is blocked by a tree! Under the tree lies a dead mouse. The educator sees his well-planned lesson vanish into thin air. The thoughts and minds of the children are occupied with the dead mouse for the rest of the day. The event was, he writes, "the pedagogy of the dead mouse," which is the pedagogy that deals with the unplanned and how teachers can meet the unexpected (Granath 1988, pp. 50–51).

The story by Mats Granath has some similarities to the story above. In both stories, we meet children who fall into a state of wonder. Another similarity is that both the father and the educator have a plan and are heading towards a goal. To have a plan and to reach a goal is important in many educational situations. Sometimes, however, the focus on the aim of the educational session may prevent a teacher from seeing the potential for wonder along the way and what this could evoke. In Granath's article, the extraordinary event struck the children with wonder in the face of the mystery of life and death materialized in the form of a dead mouse. As grown-ups, it might be easier to recognize the wonder and feel astonishment at the fact that the universe and all its stars could arise. A dead mouse or a snail creeping over a stone might not create the same surprise and amazement. Generally, children may be better than adults at being in a state of wonder. But there is also something about the situations in these stories that can evoke wonder. The sensitivity for the surroundings might be sharpened when a child is out late at night or walking in the woods. A person might see and hear more attentively compared to when he or she is in a safe and well-known environment.

The following elaboration is based on the assumption that the children and the adults in these two stories could exemplify two different ways of wonder and wondering which could express two different ways of relating to the world. I am going to examine this assumption by applying the philosophy of Martin Buber, and his description of the human being's twofold attitudes toward the world. From a philosophical, anthropological approach, he suggests that we relate to the world either through an I and It relationship or an I and Thou relationship. Examining these attitudes might be helpful concerning understanding the difference between "falling into wonder" or "being in wonder" and "wondering about something," which indicate different ways of positioning oneself. Moreover, I think these two different relationships could also nurture reflections on questions about meaning and attachment to the world. They can help to understand why an instrumental orientation provides detachment and distance as opposed to a dialogical relationship where one is in touch with the world in a different way.

ON TWO DIFFERENT WAYS OF RELATING TO THE WORLD

The philosopher Martin Buber (1878–1965) is well-known for his book *I and Thou* (1923/2004) and his epistemological distinction between I and Thou and I and It. To man, according to Buber (2004), the relation to the world is twofold. The sphere of the I and It constitutes all mental acts that are directed toward an object: "I perceive something, I am sensible of something, I imagine something, I will do something, I feel something. I think something" (Buber, 2004, p. 12). The educators in our context wish to teach something to the children. The acts involve a sort of mastery, namely the human capacity to extract knowledge from the constitution of things to separate objects from objects, and to analyze them. An I and It relationship involves acts such as describing, naming, classifying, and defining an object and its boundaries to systematically relate objects to each other (ibid., 11–14). These activities are ways of controlling and organizing a detached world. In many ways, the description fits how academic knowledge is considered and presented. Buber would not say that this is wrong and should be avoided (Kristiansen, 2013). He thinks that people live large parts of their lives in an I and It relationship and see the world as an object for use and misuse. Problems only arise when the attitude becomes too dominant. He suggests there is also another way of relating to the world, namely by saying the primary words *I* and *Thou*. He writes: "Primary words do no describe something that might exist independently of them but being spoken they bring about existence" (Buber, 2004, p. 11). It is interesting to notice that in this sphere, there are no activities such as sorting, naming, or comparing, but the person is directly confronting what is in front of him or her. The relation to the Thou is direct: "No system of ideas, no foreknowledge, and fancy intervene between I and Thou. . . . Every means is an obstacle. Only when every means has collapsed does the meeting come about" (Buber, 1974, p. 17). In the meeting, the speaker has nothing. Buber writes:

> When Thou is spoken, the speaker has no thing for his object. For where there is a thing there is another thing. Every it is bounded by others; it exists only through being bounded by others. But when Thou is spoken, there is no thing.

> Thou has no bounds. When Thou is spoken, the speaker has no thing; he has indeed nothing. But he takes his stand in relation. (Buber, 2004, p. 12)

In a mutual relationship, there is a shared presence where what we encounter is emerging in its own appearance. At the moment, it stands for itself—in its uniqueness—and is determined based on the mutuality that has occurred. Levinas writes about the I and Thou relation that it "consists in confronting a being external to oneself, i.e., one which is radically other, and to recognize it as such" (Levinas, 1967, p. 138). This does not mean, he continues, to have an idea of something which is appropriate to the I and It relation. What is important is not thinking about the other. To say Thou is an immediate contact, "an appeal which does not posit an object" (ibid., p. 138). In the I and It relations the person will relate to the world as it appears in his or her experience, analyses, judgments or his and her way of doing things (Friedman, 1976, p. 68). In the I and Thou encounter, the world is "external to oneself" and is "existing for itself" (Buber, 1988, p. 52) and it speaks to you.

According to Buber the world of I and Thou relations includes three spheres: the life with men as presented above, with nature, and with spiritual beings (Buber, 2004, p. 13). Regarding the life with nature, a tree, for instance, could be considered as an It. The tree could be measured, classified, and put in a numerical relation. However, the tree could also be "seized by the power of exclusiveness" (Buber, 1974, p. 14). A moment can arise when the wholeness of the tree is "bodied over against me and has to do with me, as I with it—only in a different way" (Buber, 2004, p. 15). But can a human being encounter a tree? A tree cannot speak, and how can this relationship be mutual? In an afterword to the book *I and Thou* (1923/2004), Buber admits that there have been questions regarding whether it is possible to have an I and Thou meeting with a tree. Even if a tree or a flower cannot respond in the same way a person can, he does not think this means that there will be no reciprocity at all. The tree in its unity and wholeness discloses itself to the glance of the one who says Thou (Buber, 2004, p. 95). Although the meeting will not have the same qualities as a person—person relationship, something dynamic is happening. The tree stands out and has to do with me.

The world of relations also includes life with spiritual beings. Similarly to the two other spheres, the encounter and how the person relates is the essential. A basic assumption in Buber's thinking is that there is a close connection to God in the relation to one's fellow man (Buber, 2004, p. 93). To address the concrete other as a *Thou* represents an encounter with the Eternal Thou (Mendes-Flohr, 1986). Buber was influenced by Hasidism, a Jewish religious movement (Buber, 1978, pp. 213–16). A basic idea is that genuine relations converge into the Eternal Thou and in our lives—the I and Thou meeting—brings life and sanctity to daily tasks and routine. This insight, according to

Alexandre Guilherme (2011), reminds us that the divine is present everywhere and that religion and the concrete everyday life are intrinsically interconnected (Guilherme, 2011).

In Buber's thinking it is the meeting that is essential. The present Thou, whether it is a person, a cat—or even a dead mouse—is a window to the Eternal Thou. The term "present" (German "präsenz") has a double meaning. The concept can be interpreted as presence, meaning closeness, nearness, and proximity, but can also be linked to time– the present or our time. In this context, time does not mean clock time or mechanical time but time as "filled present" (Buber, 2004, p. 18). The dynamic content is defined in light of what stands right before the person, whether this is another person, an animal, or a tree.

In contrast to if the content had been decided in advance based on previous experiences, definitions, and analyses, the I and Thou meeting happens here and now. In the present moment, for a person who is aware and listening, the Thou touches and has to do with her or him in a significant way.

ETHICAL AND RELIGIOUS DIMENSIONS: A CALL FOR HUMANITY

The idea that there is a religious dimension inherent in everyday life bears similarities to the thinking of the Danish theologian and philosopher Knud E. Løgstrup's and his outlines of the spontaneous life utterances (see chapter 7 in this book). Trust is an example of a spontaneous life utterance that is located in the interhuman life. A characteristic of trust, like other interhuman phenomenon, is that it is not subject to a human determination or decision. Trust is given and cannot be insisted on or ordered. The ethical demand that is embodied in the phenomenon itself is directed toward taking care of the life that is given in the relationship (Løgstrup, 1966, pp. 194–95). There are other similarities between Buber and Løgstrups's thinking. They both underline the spontaneous and immediate and that there are dimensions in human life that is beyond the control of human beings. According to Buber (2004), a person doesn't choose or decide when he or she is met, addressed, or touched by something or someone. He writes: "The Thou meets me through grace—it is not found by seeking." (Buber, 2004, p. 17). What happens cannot be attributed to the person's efforts, but occurs by grace. Another similarity is how the realisations both of the spontaneous life utterances and of the immediate meeting is connecting human beings to the world around them. The spontaneous and immediate responses create bonding and relationships (Løgstrup, 1975). However, Buber and Løgstrup start their philosophical analysis from different theoretical approaches. Løgstrup's approach is a phenomenological analysis, while Buber's approach is philosophical anthropology and has an anthropological foundation. In Løgstup's thinking, the ethical demand inherent in the interhuman phenomenon is more explicitly formulated. There is a sort of demand in Buber's description of the encounter, but it is more vague. It is an encouragement to take part, to be active, and to bond. However, using a phrase like 'a person is addressed' could give associations to a narrow moral category in the sense that people thereby are responsible for some judgmental body. Buber's perspective seems to be more existential with a sharper focus on how human beings encounter and respond to the world in general. Thus, phrases such as 'to be addressed' and 'a world that is reaching out to human beings' give associations to a dynamic world that calls to people and their willingness to take part and to fulfil themselves creatively and spiritually. It could be characterised as a call for humanity. By responding to the call, by acting, one is invited to create something together. Buber writes:

> We respond to the moment, but at the same time we respond on its behalf, we answer for it. A newly created concrete reality has been laid in our arms; we answer for it. A dog has looked at you, you answer for its glance, a child has clutched your hand, you answer for its touch. . . . (Buber, 1978, p. 17)

There is no recipe for how the response should be carried out, but the response should neither be solely intellectual nor emotional. The call is aimed at the whole human being and entreats us to respond in a wholehearted and dedicated way. According to Buber (1966), the true norm does not only demand the person's obedience, but his or her whole self—it requires the person's humanity (Buber, 1966, p. 2). Although there is no recipe for how to respond to the call, the response involves the wholeness of man. In the mutual community that arises, something human is realized.

The quotation above describes a world in which humans themselves cannot choose when it suits them to be addressed, touched, and called to act responsibly. Buber places man in a world that is reaching out to human beings, a world that speaks and calls on man for "company" and dialogue. To meet the dog's gaze, to hold on the child's hand, is to respond to a call that invites to responsibility and fellowship. In the community that arises, the humane is expressed. It is a community with a world that is not only exclusive to humans, but also includes animals and nature. One might say that it is life itself—through what surrounds us here and now—that calls for our awareness, our humanity and participation.

In the following, based on insights from Buber's thinking, I will examine what types of wonder are found in the two stories. First, the inquisitive kind where one is wondering *about* something. Second, the marvelling kind, wondering *at* something, as a more spontaneous state described as to fall in into a state of wonder, to be affected by wonder, or *to be in wonder*.

TO WONDER ABOUT SOMETHING AND TO BE IN WONDER

In the first story, we meet a father who has a plan and an aim for the journey, namely to show his son the wonder and majesty of the universe. Many parents would approve of this aim. Most of us would agree that the universe is something to wonder about and that we seldom take the time to do so. It is the father who organized the journey, and he knows the final stop. Throughout the story, he appears to be in control, and does not seem to deviate from this plan. When they arrive at the meadow, he lifts his son and starts to name the stars. Like many teachers before him, he is eagerly demonstrating his knowledge of the matter. At this point, his son has already lost interest. The father is approaching "his" wonder very much in an I and It relation. Another approach could have been to create a space where the starry sky could "speak" to both.

Unlike the father's approach, where wonder is a planned event, the son is discovering a lot of small surprises along the route. Compared to the father's brilliant and magnificent object of wonder, the son's discoveries in the surrounding environment are almost invisible and not exactly breathtaking. A snail creeping over a stone creates wonder. The father's "wonder" is ahead of them. His gaze towards the future goal might prevent him from discovering together with the son the wonders of the universe that could be found along the route.

A similar awareness is shown by the children who are taking a walk with their teacher. Something suddenly lights up and approaches the children; the dead mouse is lying there right in front of them on the trail. In a Buber-inspired way, we could say that they are facing a reality that discloses itself to them. They are called by something in the situation, and in the moment, a feeling of astonishment and compassion might arise. The children perceive the mouse in its entirety; the colour, the size, and the damage that is united in this event. The mouse is present in a single whole, and it has to do with them (Buber, 2004, p. 14). Here and now, the "Gestalt" or the wholeness of what they concretely encounter is reaching out and challenging the individual as an active person.

A dead mouse might not be the best example or starting point considering a discussion about mutuality. However, a prerequisite for the dynamic in an I and Thou relationship is that the Thou "has been set at a distance, more precisely, has become an independent opposite" (Buber, 1988, p. 50).

This characteristic will have implications for the understanding of a state of wonder in the frame of an I and Thou relationship, even if a community arose between the I and the Thou that indicates not a kind of same-meltdown or dissolution of the I and the Thou into one subject. In a conversation with Carl Rogers, Buber is using the term "detached presence" to underline the idea that even if two persons feel a high degree of closeness and have a particular situation in common, there could be structures that create distance. Such structures could be age, different roles, different perspectives (Buber, 1965). An experience of being in wonder could evoke a robust mystical experience and a feeling of unity, for instance, with God or with nature. In light of the dialogue with Carl Rogers, an interpretation could be that the Thou continues to exist for itself and maintains the otherness. This aspect makes it possible to take care of another characteristic of dialogue, according to Buber, namely the possibility of being surprised (Buber, 1965, p. 178). In the I and Thou relationship, the person meets what is independent and different. Thus, it involves the possibility of becoming surprised. In a dialogue, the person mentally "reaches over there" to the other, but simultaneously keeps his or her ground in the relationship. Buber denotes this with the term Umfassung (Embracing). Here, the other's differentness is maintained while a connection is established. In the act of inclusion, the person experiences two things simultaneously, Buber writes, "first that he is limited by otherness, and second that he receives grace by being bound to the other" (Buber, 1978, p. 101).

Therefore, to wonder in an I and Thou relationship is not about losing oneself or disappearing in a mystical event. Quite the contrary; the moment is grounded in concrete reality and cannot be perceived as an isolated and mystical event. These moments are closely related to the everyday life of people and are latent possibilities in their specific environment. What is crucial is people's relationships with the world that surrounds them, to be in touch with, and to be actively participating in this reality, such as growing their garden and grooming their livestock. Mental confinement to specific theories, or adopting an instrumental mindset, can prevent humans from entering what Buber calls "living connections" with the beings and things whose lives we are supposed to take part in, like they in ours. The soul becomes dry and barren if we do not "day by day, offer these small meetings that we are due to them" (Buber, 1963, p. 49, my translation). To be responsible, and to answer, expresses an entrance into life. The humanizing moment is found not *above* but *in* life and participation.

THE COMMUNITY IS A SHARED APPRECIATION

There is a sense of sadness involved in the story about the father and son's journey. Despite the father's efforts, purpose, and well-planned trip, he fails to arouse his son's sense of wonder for something he appreciates. Both father and son are wondering at the universe, but they are gazing in different directions and are not able to share each other's appreciation.

There could be various reasons for this lack of shared appreciation. One might be the father's eagerness to start naming the stars above them. Such an act could contribute to the creation of distance between father and son. The son might be impressed by his father's knowledge, or it could feel instructive and overwhelming. By these actions, the father risks shadowing the phenomena instead of taking a step aside and letting the event itself "speak." By taking a step back, it migt have been possible for the two of them to share a moment of co- attention while looking in the same direction.

In the chapter by Rita Nordström-Lytz called *Presence as Silence in the Educational Encounter* (2012), she describes a community between a father and his little son. Even if a relationship between a grown-up and a child cannot be mutual in the sense that a child cannot be able to throw himself across and experience from "over there," they are sharing a moment of great fun. The story is from a novel by Henry D. McHenry, where he describes how he experienced a moment of immediate presence together with his son. On a rainy afternoon, while sitting at his computer working on a manuscript, he hears an excited voice from outside the house. His young son is running around on the grass, soaking wet and shouting for joy. Although the father at first merely watches his son for a while, he then joins the boy, whose face is alight with happiness and excitement, and they share the joy of rain and running in this conversation:

> "I don´t know what came over me—I was just running around like crazy in the yard . . . "
>
> "I know," I said.
>
> "What?" he asked breathlessly.
>
> "*Rain-running happiness.*" (Nordström-Lytz, 2012, p. 85)

Nordström-Lytz thinks this short description can serve as an illustration of presence in an educational encounter, a momentary setting when preconceived opinions and attitudes are set aside. The parties involved "having nothing" as opposed to having something—for instance, a plan—a concept that could emphasize the open registering of speaking and listening to that which occurs here and now. She continues:

> This brief story seems to illustrate the "having nothing"—character of presence, namely the openness towards what is to come—and capturing this precise moment. . . . It is the turning to the other, like Buber says, attuning one´s awareness, not into a no-where but the person(s) encountering in the actual upcoming concrete situation. (Nordström-Lytz, 2012, p. 85)

It is an immediate response to the other person as well as to the exact location. Openness towards anything to come includes having an attitude of seeing-as-a-wonder, which opens up for one´s creativity. When having nothing fixed or planned, every opportunity is open and available.

The encounter establishes a co-creation between the parties and the situation involved. The rain, the splashing, the dancing, the father and the son—all are captured by a present shared moment. Although the relationship is not fully reciprocal, it is the joint participation that seems decisive.

TOWARD THE END: SOME EDUCATIONAL REFLECTIONS

Insights from Buber's thinking has revealed that there can be two ways of relating to the world when wondering: wondering about something or falling into a state of wonder and being in wonder. Only the latter approach brings human beings in touch with the world in a dialogical sense. There are some educational aspects which I want to reflect upon a bit more toward the end.

Normally, teaching and learning happen inside the school building. The school has a particular organization, a curriculum, and some defined goals for the various teaching activities. The situations in the aforementioned stories all take place outside the school. Even so, there are some interesting teaching and learning implications. According to Michael Bonnet (2009), it is a general phenomenon that we are alle claimed by places: "no action is possible in the absence of place, nor any thought, including that of sense of self. They all presuppose a milieu of prompts and claims" (Bonnet, 2009, p. 5). He continues: "It might be argued that finding oneself in a strange environment might heighten one's senses of self . . . and different places/neighbourhoods/situation prompt—call for—different responses" (ibid., 5). While the classroom and a school are constructed for learning, the children in the three stories are outdoors exposed to the "real" and to the complexity of the environment.

In additional to being outdoors, the persons are moving; they are walking, dancing and pointing. Jan Masschelein has developed a pedagogy where the gaze is connected to movement. He invites the students to city walks in foreign places in order to help them to be more attentive, since the gaze is itself bound to a perspective and a particular position. According to Masschelein

(2010), when walking the road, the walking "commands us" to displace our gaze so that we can see differently. Walking is about being-out-position and "to be there—in the present—in such a way that the present can present itself to me" (Masschelein, 2010, p. 48). The pedagogy that Masschelein develops underlines the risky, insecure and challenging, as opposed to being in a position of control and being the master of the situation. In addition, it could stimulate wondering in two ways: First, the possibility to see in a different way and to wonder about it. Second, because of strengthening the awareness of the surroundings and the situation, it could encourage people to engage and to take part.

To wonder and to be in wonder are actions which shed light on some educational moments that have a tendency not to dominate the educational agenda. One reason is already mentioned. The various claims of learning effectiveness and the emphasis on the teaching results might lead to less attention toward slower learning processes, such as wondering, where the result is in the open and cannot be given beforehand. An overly strong focus on the teaching aims and results could also contribute to less space for student initiative and wondering questions, outdoors, as well as in the classroom.

The father in the first story has his mind oriented toward the goal of the walk and his eyes are looking up at the majestic starry sky. Because of this, the kind father forgets to listen and be aware of his son's experiences along the road. Expressed in a more metaphorical way, his upward attention prevents him from being in touch with the world around him and to see and listen to all the mysteries along the road his son is attentive to. But even if the father in his eagerness to show the son the majesty of the universe fails to be attentive to the world around, he does something interesting. He points towards the stars and by doing so draws the child's attention to the wonder and mystery. A sense of wonder, and situations that could create wonder, are normally not high on the school's agenda. By pointing, the father is directing the child's gaze while the autonomy of the child is maintained.

The roles of the grown-ups are interesting in the three stories. In the stories about the dead mouse and the father and son dancing together in the rain, the action of the child also affects the authority of the adult and the control of the situation. Buber presents to us a world that is reaching out to human beings, a world that is not disenchanted and without meaning. It is a world that calls to human beings for response and participation, and according to Buber's inspiration from Hasidism, to perfect it. Normally it is the teacher who brings the teaching material in front of the children. In the three stories, it is the children who "bring the content to the table" and the children invite the teacher to take part in their wondering. A community of wondering is established. However, there is a distinction between the children, who are immediately gripped by astonishment, and the teacher. She or he enters the situation some minutes later, first listening to what the children are saying and then participating in the wondering conversation. In terms of the two positions—to wonder about something and to be in wonder—the teacher represents a scholarly way of wondering very much in line with to wonder *about* something. The teacher has a double consciousness; on the one hand being fully engaged in the conversation, while on the other hand also being aware of her or his role as a teacher. In the latter case, the teacher wishes to participate in the ongoing conversation and so invites the children to step out of the existential position and enter an explorative stage.

The act of wondering implies a relationship between a person and the world. The action may be directed from the person toward the world or—the other way round—from the world to the person. If instrumental thinking is dominant, where the gaze is fixed on the target and on the methods of reaching this goal, it can lead to less sensitivity toward the situation and the interhuman dimensions involved. In Buber's description, it is life itself that calls people to act and to participate and not to be an observer. Participation involves responsibility, and the relationship brings existence and life. It is in this life-giving and concrete relationship that our humanity is nurtured. According to the Buber scholar Maurice Friedman (1978), "our age is seen as the most homeless of all because of the loss of an image of the world. . . . And a sense of community" (Friedman, 1978, pp. xix and xx). The modern man has turned him- or herself into an onlooker without any feeling of belonging to the world. Human beings, Buber writes, has lost "the unconscious humanity of being part of participation and partaking" (Buber, 1978, p. 87). To fall into wonder may be a way to restructure a lost connection and improve participation. Something "lights up" and we respond to it. Being in wonder, is a humanizing moment found not beyond life but within life—in everyday participation. Later, we start wondering about what happened.

Buber presents the reader to a world where the divine is hidden, but present in immediate encounters. The implicit religious dimension indicates that wonder and wondering are natural and integrated aspects of everyday life—often in terms of wondering about something, but in an exclusive way in the immediate I and Thou relationship. The father in the first story is pointing towards the stars and beyond the everyday life of human beings. By this he is directing the gaze of his son toward the infinite universe. But his son had already discovered the universe in a snail creeping over a stone and a blade of grass swaying tin the wind. Even if the encounters happen in a short period of time, they might nurture a sense of wonder that could be present as a soft echo when the father and son, hand in hand, return home for dinner.

REFERENCES

Bonnett, M. (2010). Schools as places of unselving: an educational pathology? Paper given at the conference "Perspectives on Pedagogy and Place," The University of Oslo, Nov. 12–13, 2009.

Buber, M. (1963). *Menneskets vej efter den chassidiske lære*. Oslo: Aschehoug.

Buber, M. (1966). *Møde med mennesker*. København: Hasselback kulturbibliotek.

Buber, M. (1978). *Between Man and Man*. New York: Macmillan Publishing.

Buber, M. (1988). *The Knowledge of Man: Selected Essays*. Atlantic Highlands: Humanities Press International, Inc.

Buber, M. (2004). *I and Thou*. London, New York: Continuum.

Friedman, M. (1976). *Martin Buber: The Life of Dialogue*. Chicago and London: The University of Chicago Press.

Friedman, M. (1978). Introduction to Between Man and Man. In M. Buber (1978). *Between Man and Man*. New York: Macmillan Publishing.

Giddens, A. (1992). *The Consequences of Modernity*. Cambridge: Polity Press.

Guilherme, A. (2011). God as Thou and Prayer as Dialogue: Martin Buber's Tools for Reconciliation. In Sophia, published online: 03 November 2011.

Gur-Ze'ev, I. (2005). Beyond Postmodern Feminist Critical Pedagogy—Toward a Diasporic Pedagogy of Counter-Education. In I. Gur-Ze'ev (ed.) *Critical Theory and Critical Pedagogy Today: Toward a New Critical language in Education* (pp. 160–92). Haifa: University of Haifa.

Granath, M. (1988). *Den døda musens pedagogik*. Debattserien nr.1, pp. 50–51.

Kristiansen, A. (2015). Educational challenges in the shadow of instrumentalism. In S. Hillen and C. Aprea (eds.) *Instrumentalism in Education—Where is Bildung left?* (pp. 117–30). Göttingen: Waxman Verlag.

Kristiansen, A. (2013). Experiences of silence in education: Some reflections. In red. H. Elvstrand, K. Forslund Fykedal, M.Samuelsson, R. Thornberg, *Lärares etik och professionella arbete: Skolan som moralisk praktik*. Linköping: Linköping University.

Levinas, E. (1976). Martin Buber and the theory of knowledge. In ed. Paul Arthus Schilpp and Maurice Friedman, *The Philosophy of Martin Buber.* The library of living philosophers, vol. XII, pp. 133–50. Cambridge University Press: London.

Løgstrup, K. E. (1966). *Kunst og etik*. København: Gyldendal.

Løgstrup, K. E. (1975). *Den etiske fordring*. København: Gyldendal.

Masschelein, J. (2010). E-ducation the gaze: the idea of a poor pedagogy. Ethics and Education, Vol. 5, No. 1, pp. 43–53.

McHenry, Henry D., Jr. (1997). Education as an Encounter: Buber's Pragmatic Ontology. *Educational Theory*, Vol. 47, Issue 3: 341–357.

Mendes-Flohr, P. (1986). *Marin Buber's conception of God.* Erstratto da: Teologia Filsofica E. Filosofia Della Religione. Perugia: Editrice Benucci. *Educational Theory* 47:3, pp. 341–57.

Nordström-Lytz, Rita (2012). Presence as Silence in the Educational Encounter. In ed. Henny Fiskå Hägg and Aslaug Kristiansen, *Attending to Silence: Educators and Philosophers on the Art of Listening*, pp. 81–92. Kristiansand: Portal Academic.

Stark, U. (2016) *When Dad Showed Me the Universe*. Gecko Press. White paper: St.melding nr. 30 Kultur for læring (2003–2004).

Chapter 8

Listening to the Silence of Wonder and Reconquering Spaces for Human Flourishing

Ortheil's Novel Die Erfindung des Lebens *and Lightart in the Corona Crisis*

Claudia Welz

Hanns-Josef Ortheil's award-winning novel *Die Erfindung des Lebens* (*The Invention of Life,* 2009), which has autobiographical elements, can be read as a *Bildungsroman* describing the interrelation between education and character development, between the discovery of the world and a language in which the protagonist can express himself. The author, whose story is the topic of the book, could not speak as a child. He was born after WWII as the fifth child of his parents, who had lost four sons during the war. This unbearable loss muted his mother. The novel narrates the surprising process in which the boy and his mother regain speech despite serious traumatization. For years, they only communicated through silent gestures and looks, through daily rituals and music. Their transformation is linked to moments of wonder that are not only eye-opening, but also mouth-opening for them in triggering speech. However, before they experienced 'the silence of wonder,' they had to stand the ambiguity of silences that were mostly painful and only sometimes peaceful. The metamorphosis of the mother and her child is closely related to the opening up of spaces for human flourishing which they first had to recapture and reconquer in times of crisis: landscapes, cultural settings, the private home, churches, and prayer rooms.

Based on an analysis of this novel, I will, in a first step, explore the aesthetical, ethical, and spiritual dimensions of a meaningful 'being-in-the-world,' of 'being-with-others,' and of 'being-oneself-in-relation-to-the-divine.' Special attention will be paid to experiences of that which makes life worth living and turns us into creatures that are open to encounters leading us beyond ourselves, to the other or the wholly Other. Due to God's unavailability or transcendence, we do not always have direct access to that which has called us into existence and sustains our lives. In exploring Ortheil's descriptions of the 'wonder' that changed his life, I want to trace the movements in which the 'beyond' can enter into our everyday lives and come close to us. The question that interests me particularly in this context is twofold: What does it mean to 'listen' to the silence of wonder in which we are ready to receive the other or wholly Other, and how can we attend to the 'call' that is implicit in a wondrous situation, relation, or moment?

In a second step, I will contextualize the insights extracted from Ortheil's novel by relating them to theological, phenomenological, psychological, and hermeneutical approaches to the key terms of this paper: 'listening' and 'silence.' I will argue that we can access silence through its effect on the listener: its resonance. Hence, it becomes necessary to clarify what it means to listen to resounding silence. In regard to God's 'silence' and 'listening,' I will discuss suggestions by Rachel Muers and Nelle Morton; in regard to interhuman silence, the work of Don Ihde and Bernhard Waldenfels, Günter Bader, Dan Bar-On, Irene Levin, and James Risser will come into focus.

I will then, in a third step, return to Ortheil's novel in order to learn more about spaces, conditions, and practices promoting or obstructing human flourishing. Evaluating his positive and negative examples, supplemented by the presentation of a contemporary performance of lightart in the corona crisis, I will finally draw conclusions in regard to practices in education and healthcare that might make human beings more attuned to what they are 'called' to. In other words, I will show in what ways Ortheil's novel is relevant for a re-humanizing reform of professional practices.

1. ORTHEIL ON LISTENING TO THE SILENCE OF WONDER

The first-person narrator in Ortheil's novel looks back on his life. His retrospective account begins with childhood memories. Together with his mother and father, he lived in Cologne. He describes their life together as a small circle of three human beings who basically remained isolated from the world outside. They lived "in a kind of close-lipped secret society (*in einer Art verschwiegenem Geheimbund*) with only the most necessary external relations"

(Ortheil, 2011, 38). The life of the family followed firm rules and took place "in a great silence (*in einer großen Stille*): it was the uncanny postwar-silence of the fifties, which seemed to originate from a great exhaustion and in which every sound, every voice, and every tone was perceived perfectly well" (ibid.). To the boy, the surroundings were like a "noiseless zone" (ibid., 39) where people usually spoke quietly or even whispered on the streets and where there was no radio and no television. The boy tried to identify the sounds of the street by lying on the floor with closed eyes in front of an open window in his parents' apartment and harkening intensely. He listened to footsteps and voices as if they constituted a piece of music. Thereby, he trained his sense of hearing and learned to differentiate between sounds and tones (see ibid., 40).

He experienced silence in ambiguous ways. On the one hand, he suffered from the silence of muteness, of speechlessness. He, the boy who could not speak, was "the mute [. . .] image of the misery" that had befallen his parents (ibid., 42). He hated the "completely silent moments" in which he felt that all gazes were directed at him, when nobody spoke, but everyone expected him to do something he could not do (ibid., 49). It was terrible for him when other children's mothers called him a 'poor boy' because of his lack of spoken language and said to each other that one must be grateful for having a healthy kid (see ibid., 50). On the other hand, he experienced silence as something wonderful—not as a thing or an entity, but rather as an opening in which wonder in the sense of marvel can change everything: the whole situation, the whole life of a person, including him- or herself.

In what follows, I will analyze key scenes in Ortheil's novel where the silence of wonder creates spaces for human flourishing. In particular, I will focus on three different dimensions of wonder, namely (1) spirituality, the sense of and search for something greater than oneself, where wonder not just surfaces as 'the dearest child of faith,' as an old proverb has it, but also as an entrance point for the sacred, the divine or transcendent, even in places where one would not expect it; (2) ethics, here understood as the sphere of human action and interaction, where wonder is experienced in the form of a 'real' and deep encounter between human beings whose relation to each other is transformed; and (3) aesthetics, here defined as a discipline dealing with αἴσθησις (*aisthēsis*: sense perception) in general and artistic expression in particular, where wonder appears in various forms of beauty mediated by music, poetry, or visual art.

1.1 Spirituality: Attending To God's Presence

Wonder in the context of spirituality is not limited to certain religious traditions. Rather, it can 'break into' our everyday lives as a surprise. Wonder is related to a 'beyond' in the sense that we cannot control, possess, or dispose of it. It is not something that is 'in our hands,' so to say. It comes 'from outside' the reach of human possibilities, and it refers us to 'larger hands' that can hold, sustain, and protect not just our lives, but the whole planet or even the entire universe.

My approach to the spiritual dimensions of the silence of wonder is phenomenological by focusing on the ways in which these dimensions are experienced or 'given' to consciousness. As they are 'about' something which eludes comprehension and withdraws from perception, it is only in a metaphorical sense that we can speak of 'listening' to the silence of wonder. It lies in the nature of silence that, strictly speaking, there is nothing to be 'heard'—at least not acoustically. Thus, in 'listening' to the silence of wonder, we need more than our physical ears in order to really 'receive' that which cannot be 'heard' via ordinary audition. But how, then, can we get in touch with the Holy if it is defined as a wholly Other? To anticipate my point: we are touched by it in ways that exceed the grasp of our senses and our intellect, even if we combine all our mental capacities in a concerted effort. It belongs to the task of an existential hermeneutics (see Welz, 2018) to unearth the meaning of the 'silence of wonder,' which is not written down in any text, but may be found between the lines, at the margins of consciousness, in real life.

The protagonist in Ortheil's novel remembers how he and his mother went to a nearby chapel every second day. They only spent some minutes there, but these minutes left an indelible impression. There was a niche for prayer with a painting of Mary and many candles. Every time the two kneeled in front of this image, something peculiar happened to the boy: the more he concentrated on the image, the more silent the church room around them seemed to be. Only the finest sounds could be heard, such as the crackling of the burning candles. And the more silent everything became, the more clearly and mightily the image of Mary radiated. This had a calming effect on the boy, whose gaze was fixed upon the face of beautiful Mary as if he were hypnotized and stunned in a "hypnosis of silence (*Hypnose der Stille*)" (Ortheil, 2011, 54).

In this state, he began to pray. He did so not by imagining or thinking of certain words, but rather by listening to how the praying commenced in him by itself.[1] The boy's prayer began when the well-known prayers came to his mind. Ortheil here speaks of *einfallen,* which literally means 'falling in': the words fell into the mind of the praying boy. He then silently spoke the prayers in his mind from the beginning to the end. The narrator admits that the intensity of his prayer also was due to the fact that he was kneeling next to his mother who prayed with the utmost devotion, tension, and concentration, incessantly looking at Mary, as if she was begging for a conversation, a response, or at least a little clue. The boy felt that this private ritual had something urgent to it, so he assumed that it was about life or death. He interpreted prayer as a "stepping in front of God" (*Hintreten vor Gott*) during which one tells him what has happened, an occasion on which one speaks some verses, and finally asks for God's blessing (ibid., 55). Moreover, prayer was, for him, also a matter of looking back and pondering whether he had acted correctly in a certain situation.

While praying, the boy felt he was in the presence of God. God is described with the help of visual metaphors. God is "the highest and most radiant instance" (*die höchste und strahlendste Instanz*) before which the human being's "small life" (*kleines Leben*) retracts and changes "into a wide, open, great life" (*in ein weites, offenes, großes Leben*) (ibid., 56). It is noteworthy that God is silent while this amazing transformation of human life takes place. Divine presence is, as it were, the 'catalyst' that makes possible the widening, broadening, and growth of human life. For the boy, a tiny little hole in the vault above the main altar in Cologne Cathedral, through which the sunlight streams into the room, was the "bolthole" (*Schlupfloch*) of God's infinity (ibid., 57). While there is no mention of a speaking God, the boy liked the singing and praying of the congregation. Inwardly and quietly, he participated in the praise of God—with the effect that he no longer felt secluded from other people. In the Cathedral, he belonged to the community, was part of the group, and no one claimed that he was a "poor child" (*armes Kind*), for in the Cathedral, there were only children of God (*Gotteskinder*); the archbishop called all believers *Gotteskinder,* which was "the real redemption" (*eigentliche Erlösung*) for the boy, one of the most beautiful states to be in (ibid., 60).

In his reflection on the services in Cologne Cathedral, Ortheil concludes retrospectively that the ceremony had "transfigured" (*verwandelt*) those who listened to the music of the organ and the choir and looked at the slow movements and gestures of the clergymen: "In the Cathedral, I thus learned how to truly see and hear," he writes: it was "as if the powerful God poured this music into one, so that one forgot all grief and woe at least for the duration of the service" (ibid., 62). When listening attentively, the boy was in a state of supreme receptivity to the marvelous event that would bring him *coram deo,* near to God, whose presence would change everything.

1.2 Ethics: Human Action and Interpersonal Encounters

Ethics, broadly understood as a theory that deals with the (pre-)conditions, norms, and limits of human (inter)action, either in general or applied to specific questions, surfaces in Ortheil's novel insofar as Ortheil gives an account of interpersonal encounters and determined interventions that have made a difference for the protagonist and improved his situation. While he was mocked, ridiculed or interrogated at school without having been able to respond in any appropriate way, he was elsewhere welcomed warmly—not only in church, but also in a very profane place: a restaurant that was located on his way home from school. He once sneaked in to the toilet and then went through the lobby where he normally stood together with his father. He was immediately served a glass of water. This wordless gesture, which came that naturally, surprised him and made him happy because it showed that he simply "belonged" there (ibid., 121). Nobody glared at him, he was allowed to be present among the men, and when he had emptied his glass, he could leave again. Since then, he returned several times on his way home. Every time, he was greeted loudly as the youngest regular guest, the men raised their glasses to him and then continued their conversations. Here he felt he had "friends" (ibid., 122).

When he later arrived in Rome in order to study at the Conservatory of music, he experienced this as "one single, huge liberation" (ibid., 452) because people in Rome just let him be, without bothering him. Here, for the first time in his life, he had the feeling of being perfectly free of pain (ibid., 453). He made friends and enjoyed the fact that no one inquired about his earlier life, his voiceless days and lonely wanderings. In Rome, it was impossible to be isolated, for even when he went around alone, he felt he was in a direct exchange and very close contact with all people and things. He experienced it physically like "an inner and outer warmth" (*eine innere und äußere Wärme*), emotional security (*Geborgenheit*), and trust (*Vertrauen*) (ibid., 496).

When he fell in love, he did not want some "loose connection or a fleeting friendship" but rather "absolute affinity, daily togetherness, the uninterrupted, intense contact" (ibid., 529). He received new strength from what he later self-critically termed the "illusion" of "an ideal symbiosis" (ibid., 528). He put intimate togetherness in the place of his earlier 'siloed' life with his parents where he enjoyed the "undivided attention for the loved others"; yet, he did not carry this "affectionate look" over to his "Roman love cocoon" (ibid., 529)—a mistake he only discovered when it was too late. Shared enthusiasm for music, literature, art, architecture, and the lightness of bohemian life came to an abrupt end. However, since it was the conjoint celebration of aesthetic enjoyment that turned the muted boy into someone who was able to speak, we need to investigate more closely the role of aesthetics in this exceptional story. As mentioned, the notion of aesthetics is derived from the Greek word for 'sense perception'—which is the basis of artistic expression and any philosophical theory judging works of art or discussing taste, imagination, and the ability of aesthetic discrimination. While aesthetics cannot be reduced to a philosophy of art, let alone to an investigation of beauty, as it can also be defined as a 'metaphysics of experience' interpreting experiences of transcendence in the midst of the immanent world we have in common (see Jørgensen 2004, 28, 39), in Ortheil's novel, aesthetics features mostly in descriptions of how the boy and his family were touched by the beauty of music, literature, and visual art.

1.3 Aesthetics: Experiencing the Beauty of Music, Literature, and Visual Art

Ortheil not only lends words to the audible and visible, but also to that which is not itself 'given' to our senses: the tacit dimension of audition and the invisible 'surplus' of vision. The boy's silent family life was radically transformed when his traumatized, muted mother one fine day began to play the piano in their apartment. She did that totally unexpectedly when her husband and son sat in the kitchen and paged through some newspapers. Suddenly, a vibrant sound came through the corridor and grew ever louder, breaking through "the walls of silence" (Ortheil 2011, 70). This strong moment "changed everything" in that the boy all at once could *sense* life, and there it was: "fresh, overwhelming, enrapturing" (ibid.). The music was "a pull" speaking of "freedom and felicity" (ibid., 71), and the boy forgot all suffering. This music appeared to be like an "exit leading outside" (*Ausweg ins Freie*) into another, better world, and in retrospect, the grown-up man labelled it a "musical miracle" (*Musikwunder*) (ibid.). On the same day, the boy started to play the piano as well, and this became his "liberation" (ibid., 77) because he had finally found a way of expressing himself. Music, this 'language' beyond words, broke open a new space of being for him.

It turned out that he had a rare talent: he could see the whole score of a musical piece in his mind's eye (ibid., 182f). One day, he witnessed how his mother regained speech in humming and singing French chansons outdoors in a smiling landscape when she thought she was alone. He wanted to go indoors and play the melody on the piano, but before he managed to do so, he saw two boys playing football, and without thinking, he shouted: *Gebt mal her!* (ibid., 218). This was the first sentence he ever spoke in his life, encouraging the boys to pass on the ball, and one of the boys kicked it to him. He was startled. Had he really spoken? They had in fact understood him! From this moment, he knew he could speak. As he learned many years later, he was a baby like others when he was born; his silence only began when he was three years old. The child's silence mirrored the mother's silence. Gradually, he managed to liberate himself from the horrible past that had muted his mother. Playing the piano was his strongest aid in the struggle against silence, and to some extent, taking notes also helped him (see ibid., 439).

When he studied at the Rome Conservatory of music, his life was an ecstasy shaped by literature, film, and concerts in beautiful, old buildings (see ibid., 475, 501). However, his career as a pianist ended abruptly when he, due to tendinitis, could not play for a whole year. He returned to his parents.

During the first weeks, he could not tolerate listening to music at all—with one exception: melancholic French chansons (see ibid., 562). Was it because they can offer a different emotional access to oneself and allow mourners to work through their loss? Slowly, he found out that writing and reading aloud were a good substitute for musical expression (see ibid., 586). What we are not told in the novel is this: Ortheil became a famous writer, scholar of German literature, and professor of creative writing at the University of Hildesheim.

While it was indeed 'the silence of wonder' that he listened to in relation to God, it was 'the word' that became the vehicle of freedom in formative I-Thou-encounters between human beings, and in aesthetical contexts, it was mostly the sound of music. Thereby, the state of 'being-in-wonder,' a state that one becomes immersed in and absorbed by without having planned so, precedes the event of 'discovering-a-wonder.' As Ortheil describes the key moments of wonder in his life, he was drawn into them in a flash. He could not help being spell-bound. It was only later that he could actively respond to these events, and he did so gracefully. These events were unforeseeable, and he could only afterwards 'wonder' about that which was given to him. He was touched deeply by that which came to him 'from outside,' turning his life 'inside out.' Wonderstruck, his life received a new meaning that expanded his previous horizon of understanding.

2. LISTENING TO RESOUNDING SILENCE

Comparing spirituality, ethics, and aesthetics as potential 'containers' of wonder, it is conspicuous that silence can be evaluated differently depending on the contexts in which it occurs. In Ortheil's novel, only the silence occurring in the relationship with God appears to be unambiguously good; by contrast, in interhuman encounters, silence seems double-barreled.

2.1 Divine Silence

Interestingly, the novel ignores divine 'silence' experienced as God's 'absence' or even 'abandonment' of those believing in him. Jesus' cry from the cross as reported in the gospel of Mark (15:34: "My God, my God, why have you forsaken me?"[2]) was echoed by the cries of thousands of victims who lost their lives in Auschwitz and elsewhere. In a post-Holocaust context, divine 'silence' has become deeply ambiguous (see Welz, 2019). The same can be said about human silence before God. As Rachel Muers (2004, 8) points out, "we encounter silences of approval, disapproval, rebellion, disquiet, contentment." She suggests that "silence is neither the absence of speech nor its equivalent"; in fact, "in going beyond all the distinctions speech can make," silence "is the best communicative 'likeness' for the God who transcends all the distinctions between created things" (ibid., 11).

Muers here draws on the motif of *imago Dei,* of humanity created in God's image (Genesis 1:26f). She places the divine-human similarity or correspondence in a context of communication that involves speech and listening. Christ, the incarnate *logos* (John 1:1), is not only a speaker but also a listener. His act of hearing, as in the conversation with his disciples on the road to Emmaus (cf. Luke 24:19–24), "disrupts and transforms attempts to talk about God" (Muer, 2004, 218). Thus, divine-human communication cannot be reduced to a one-way relation dominated by the divine Word, and, on the other hand, divine silence is not absorbed into speech. Muers's claim that God can be understood "as one who keeps a *listening* silence" (ibid., 15) seems to come fairly close to Ortheil's view. Otherwise the boy's and his mother's intense prayers addressed to God would make no sense. They presuppose that he is 'present' or at least 'within call.'

Muers (ibid., 49–53) follows Nelle Morton (1985, 41), who regards hearing as a "redemptive factor." This is not only the case insofar as God receives human speech; God's hearing is empowering also because it evokes human speech. Morton calls God "a great hearing one" who "has heard us to speech" (ibid., 60). Instead of claiming that God sometimes is silent, hidden or withdrawn and that we must wait patiently until he speaks again, Morton proposes that God is like a great listening ear that "hears without interruption" (ibid., 55). God's listening enables our transition from silence to speech.

This movement corresponds exactly to the development of the plot in Ortheil's novel. Spirituality plays a priceless role in offering a dialogic field within which the divine listener and human speakers relate to each other, taking turns at speaking and listening. If God's silence is conceptualized as the silence of the listener, it can be valued because it gives space for change and, not least, for wonder, in making human beings formulate new and unexpected thoughts. This is what happened to the boy in Cologne Cathedral, where his sadness due to repudiation was transformed into a festive feeling of being welcome: the 'poor boy' became a 'child of God.' When praying in the chapel, the God who hears was also experienced as the God who responds. Now, what about the silence kept by human beings?

2.2 Human Silence

Trauma studies provide evidence for the fact that survivors often keep silent in order to protect themselves and their loved ones from the pain of the past. Here, silence functions as an unconscious defense mechanism (see Bar-On, 1989). Yet, it may also be used as an instrument of power in order to consciously hide a secret. In both cases, the act of concealment affects the agent and his or her self-understanding: "By keeping the past event silenced, one segments a certain understanding of the past and prevents it from being seen differently as time goes on" (Levin, 2013, 195). Silence can acquire multiple meanings: it can be a form of privacy or intimacy that expresses respect, but it can also be imposed on others who lose their voice and the possibility of constructing a coherent identity (see Fivush, 2010, 90f).

In Ortheil's novel, which can be read as a trauma narrative, silence is not only a 'blank space' surrounded by words, but also a phenomenon that appears 'in language' and its 'scars': as the unsayable that simultaneously comes to the fore and disappears in gaps and erasures, evasions and negations in the grammar of the said. The silence of the boy's mother directs curious interlocutors away from the traumatic event without giving them any information. The boy's own peculiar silence originates in his mother's silence, and his biography is built around the discovery of that which muted her. It was not silence itself that revealed what happened, but rather its after-effects on the ones involved, for instance the protective habits of his father. These after-effects still bear the traces of that which evoked them. They constitute, as it were, the affective 'resonance' of the traumatizing events.

Epistemologically speaking, we have access to silence and its meaning only on two conditions: (1) if we ourselves keep the silence and know why, or (2) in the case of others keeping silent, if we know what called forth the silence and 'resounds' in it. Contexts are telling as the phenomena of our world are 'speaking' to us, while we receive their meaning through the 'resonance' they produce in us. In line with this, I will approach silence via its resonance. We can listen to resounding silence only if there remain at least some faintly noticeable, barely perceptible traces of the events that preceded the silence. Yet, what exactly does it mean to 'listen' to that which, strictly spoken, cannot be 'heard'?

Don Ihde, in his pioneering work *Listening and Voice* (1976), gives us a clue. Chapter 1 starts as follows: "The beginning of man is in the midst of *word.* And the center of word is in breath and sound, in listening and speaking" (Ihde, 2007, 3). We learn that we start *in medias res*: in the submersion in language, in air, in life. We breathe and we take in spirit—and get inspired. There is a primary listening that precedes our own speech, for we always already find ourselves within language and hear the voices of others and the sounds of things before we speak (ibid., 115f). And I would like to add that we also sense the super-sensual in absorbing the atmosphere surrounding silence. Ihde argues that listening becomes 'polyphonic' insofar as it has to attend to a duet of 'voices' in the doubled modalities of perceptual and imaginative modes: 'inner' experience (imagination) may echo or mimic, present or re-present 'outer' experience (perception) in the form of memories or fantasies. This explains why, even after he became deaf, Beethoven was able to 'hear' an entire symphony at will (ibid., 117, 119).

Ihde concentrates on auditory experience, yet in appreciating "the global character of experience" (ibid., 21) that involves all senses and the richness and fullness of experience, he concedes that we hear not only with the ears but with the whole body: sound permeates our bodily being (ibid., 44f). May the same be said of silence? Silence does not send sound waves that can move and shake us, but it may convey an impression of a situation. In my view, this impression can be compared to the sensation that a still life causes when we look at it intensely. However, the question is, of course, how the visual can be 'translated' into the auditory. Or maybe the point is that we cannot and should not try to translate, but rather attend to the specific kind of experience that each of our senses can provide. Accordingly, Ihde writes: "An inquiry into the auditory is also an inquiry into the invisible. Listening makes the invisible *present* in a way similar to the presence of the mute in vision" (ibid., 51). This implies that listening comprises what seeing does not, and vice versa.

Furthermore, we have to distinguish between 'prelinguistic' levels of meaning in language-as-signification and verbal language-as-word: "To speak, to understand, and to perceive are *meaning-acts.* But what is heard, understood, and perceived [. . .] is also taken as already pregnant with meaning" (ibid., 148). There is also a silent language of gesture and touch: the smile or the frown 'speak' as well. This means that the word and its wider significance are co-present. 'Language' in this broadest sense of the word embraces silence, and, of course, we can listen to it just as we can listen to words spoken.

In order to further clarify how the audible is related to the inaudible, and whether this corresponds to the way in which the visible is related to the invisible, let us turn to phenomenologist Bernhard Waldenfels' essay about the becoming audible of the voice: "Das Lautwerden der Stimme" (2006). Following Aristotle, Waldenfels distinguishes between sounds or noises produced by things and the voice as the manifestation of an ensouled or inspirited being (ibid., 191, referring to Aristotle, *De anima* II, 8, 420 b 5f). Moreover, Waldenfels distinguishes between the event of listening (*Hörereignis*) and the act of listening (*Hörakt*), arguing that the event is irreducible to a freely performed act of listening, since the event does not begin as an act (ibid., 195). While we can decide to listen or not to listen, we cannot willingly avoid hearing what reaches our ears. There is an originary time difference between the voice reaching our ears and our listening: "*Was* ich höre, ist stets schon ein Echo dessen, *wovon* ich als Hörer getroffen bin" (ibid., 197f). According to Waldenfels, *what* I listen to (i.e., the content of a message) is always already an echo of that *by which* I am affected as a listener (i.e., uninterpreted sound waves). We have to 'listen once more' (*Nachhören*) and try to understand in order to truly be reached by the voices or sounds we have 'heard' when registering them willy-nilly.

Another person who listens attentively may even 'listen forth' my thoughts—and in this sense, my *propria vox* is a voice that is provoked (ibid., 199f). Waldenfels's essay closes with a section entitled "Unhörbares im Hörbaren" claiming that there is something inaudible within the audible:

> Wenn die Stimme unhörbar ist, so als das *Ereignis des Lautwerdens.* Darin gleicht sie dem Blick, der als Ereignis des Sichtbarwerdens unsichtbar ist. Um die Stimme zu hören, muss ich sie in ein hörbares Etwas verwandeln, so wie ich den Blick in ein sichtbares Etwas verwandeln muss, um ihn zu sehen. (ibid., 208)

Waldenfels compares the voice to the gaze: just as the gaze that makes other things visible remains invisible, so does the voice that makes other things audible remain inaudible. Thus, in order to properly 'hear' the voice, we have to transform it into something audible, just as we have to transform the gaze into something visible in order to really 'see' it, for instance by looking into a mirror. I want to contest this point. It is not *the voice* that cannot be heard, but rather *the listening*. If we, in audition, want to find an equivalent to the gaze, the zero point and blind spot of vision, this cannot be something that has already entered the acoustic sphere; rather, it is the capacity to receive the sounds of the voice—a capacity that remains inaudible.

Waldenfels delineates the relation between sonority and silence in analogy to the relation between figure and ground: silence stands out when the sounds that we have expected to hear intermit, thereby creating a 'hole' in the auditory field (ibid., 209). Here the silence of the voice refers to an absence within presence—to the inaudible within the audible. To my mind, this is a trenchant description of what happens when we listen to resounding silence, the silence left behind by an actual voice.

Resounding silence is secondary or subordinate to sound. However, there is also another kind of silence: silence pure and simple. Günter Bader (2016, 117) has captured the difference as follows: "In der Stille bleibt das Gehör leer; nicht so bei der Resonanz." Silence is here opposed to resonance in so far as there is nothing to be heard in silence. But what is it that can 'fill' the sense of hearing, that can resound and be 'heard' in the event of resonance? Is it 'the sound of silence,' a lingering sound of words spoken or music played, the reverberation of past events whose potency first shows itself in their after-effects? If this is the case, 'silence' and 'resonance' are not only (in some sense) opposed, but also dialectically intertwined. Then these terms are not mutually exclusive, but rather in need of each other, although they also remain in tension with each other.

As Bader stresses, there are two kinds of 'resonance': one that arises through audition and another that arises through the lack of something to be heard (ibid., 120). Yet, in both cases, resonance is linked with touch (*Berührung*) and mood (*Stimmung*), which can be illustrated with the help of sounds produced by string instruments (ibid., 121). Broadly speaking, 'resonance' is the power to encroach upon the natural or social environment—not only acoustically, in reaching the ears, but also in touching the hearts of those who sense that 'something' that is in the air and feel the special atmosphere surrounding it. In any case, the 'detour' via 'resonance' is necessary if we shall be able to listen to silence at all.[3]

2.3 The Role Of The Listener

Given that silence 'as such' remains 'empty' in the sense of indeterminable, how can we get access to silence that exceeds language in being located *between* the lines or *beyond* the utterances? I have argued that it can be approached only indirectly: through the ways in which it 'resonates' in those who are exposed to it.

When approaching silence via resonance, that which resounds provides the context of understanding and gives us the key to the silence we wish to interpret. By contrast, pure or total silence remains inaccessible. This also applies to the terminal silence of death, where interpretative mediation is no longer possible. However, if there is someone who listens to another's silence, he or she might 'listen forth' what is still unsaid or yet to be said.

With reference to the work of Merleau-Ponty, Heidegger, and Gadamer, James Risser (2019, 1) points out that silence is not simply the absence of speech, but always a function of language that can generate meaning. As "a space of receptivity and reticence," Risser argues, the silence of listening "allows for meaning to appear, for something to show itself, to reveal itself, in words"; and that is why hermeneutic understanding "depends fundamentally on the rigor of uninterrupted listening" (ibid., 7). Risser focuses particularly on conversations and communicative understanding in which "the inchoate word" that is literally in a beginning and does not yet say what it wants to say can be listened forth: "This silence of the unsaid speaks along with the spoken" (ibid., 11). Ideally, listening to resounding silence invites new ways of expressing what otherwise remains 'ineffable.'

This is obvious in regard to the story Ortheil tells about his childhood: he and his mother communicated in and through silence. Without his father's considerate silence of attentive listening, he would, in all probability, not have learnt to write and speak at all, and his mother would never have opened her mouth again to say a word. The boy's father did not criticize his son, neither his wife. He did not dictate terms. He listened vigilantly, but refrained from reprimanding remarks (Ortheil, 2011, 281). The narrator's father showed deference to the vulnerable in refuting others' attempts to snoop around in their traumatic past (ibid., 422).

To sum up: Various kinds of silence can become theologically, phenomenologically, psychologically, and hermeneutically evocative in their respective contexts of communication—provided that there is a 'listener' who not only attends to words, but also senses the meaning of silence. Thus, the next question is how one can come to listen in such a way that one can understand divine and (inter-)human silences. The question of "the formation of the capacity for listening and discernment" (Muers, 2004, 15) is also a question of providing adequate frameworks for learning and leisure, in which individuals get ready to listen with utmost attention. This question brings us to the third part of this paper, which is about human flourishing, seen from the professional perspectives of education and healthcare.

3. SPACES, CONDITIONS, AND PRACTICES OBSTRUCTING OR PROMOTING HUMAN FLOURISHING

Ortheil's novel gives us examples of spaces, conditions, and practices obstructing or promoting human flourishing. In what follows, an examination of these examples will lead to recommendations regarding renewed practices in education and healthcare.

3.1 That Which Obstructs and Promotes Human Flourishing

For the first-person narrator of the novel, school was one of the places where he was "punished for being mute" (Ortheil, 2011, 126). No one was interested in what he hid behind his muteness. No one knew that he "could play the piano" and "speak with beautiful Mary" and with his four brothers in heaven (ibid.). After one more "gruesome morning at school," he went to the small chapel and poured out his heart to his celestial conversation partners (ibid., 127). As mentioned, the cause of his muteness was his mother's loss of language which, in turn, was caused by the loss of four children (ibid., 280). The cruelty of this fate had literally left her speechless and "lifeless" (*leblos*) (ibid., 436).

Another place in which the boy's development was blocked was the boarding home, where he was supposed to develop his talent for music. The leave-taking of his parents was "heartbreaking" for him (*herzzerreißend*) (ibid., 340). He was homesick and missed his familiar environment. Being away was "a painful, enormous shock" that could only be overcome with the help of the idea that this was a nightmare from which he could awake (ibid., 341). Strict rules and a well-ordered daily rhythm reigned in the boarding home and the adjacent monastery. Various tasks were scheduled for every single hour. The boy was supposed to learn a lot there, but he was bothered by the fact that he could never be on his own, not even for a minute. He was always "part of a restless, nervous and often very loud community" (ibid., 343). He was not used to the permanent physical presence of other people, and therefore, his stay became a constant flight, in search of quiet zones. His reaction was a kind of 'inner emigration.' When his teachers asked, "Johannes, do you hear me?" or made remarks like, "Johannes is, again, in his own world . . . ," he was scared because this reminded him of old days he did not want to live through again (ibid., 376).

When he played Schumann on the piano, childhood memories came to his mind: of the hours together with his mother in the apartment in Cologne, of him playing at the bank of the Rhine, of walking between man-high corn forbs together with his father on paths that belonged to them alone (ibid., 332).

When he eventually ran away from the boarding home, he felt like relaxing from the "cramp" (*Verkrampfung*) of the last months (ibid., 377). While being 'caught' in the dormitory of the boarding home, he often had a strong desire to break out, to walk outside, feel some fresh air or see an unused meadow (ibid., 371). After his escape, his father came and moved to the countryside with him. He did not reproach his son for anything, but instead accepted his decision as if he had done the right thing when he ran away (ibid., 392). The boy had an ungovernable urge to be outdoors, and he enjoyed the carefree being-underway in natural surroundings (ibid., 393).

On their way to recovery from trauma, the family planned a new domicile: a remote, idyllic, tranquil place that offered shelter for them and was inaccessible to others. It contained many small hiding spots (ibid., 298f). The house in the heights was surrounded by a paradisal garden with protective barriers of hedges and forests (ibid., 498). His mother used to read a book and drink tea at specific places. This life style contributed to her convalescence.

In addition to the family's carefully planned, fanciful refuge, certain practices and rituals became vital for the boy's survival: he withdrew to the chapel, turned to the heavens and prayed. Thereby, he could order his thoughts (ibid., 120). At the boarding school, he loved to go to church early in the morning and listen to the prayer call in Latin that was repeated every day: *Deus, in adjutorium meum intende / Domine, ad adjuvandum me festina* (God, come to my aid / Lord, rush to my rescue) (ibid., 344). The silence of the night still filled the church room and was slowly dispersed through choral singing. The day began with the effort to hit one single tone in its purity. One listened to it for a while, then one stepped out of the dark into the light and bowed down before God (ibid., 345). In this way, the early hour in the abbey church held in store some of the most wonderful moments of the day (ibid., 346).

In Rome, the young man was attracted by the many churches and rooms of silence where he, again, heard the old psalmody (ibid., 457f). Here he felt safe and intuitively prayed Psalm 23: "The Lord is my Shepherd, I lack nothing. He makes me lie down in green pastures, he leads me beside quiet waters . . ." As we shall see, this psalm was central also for his father.

3.2 Recommendations Regarding a Renewed Practice in Education and Healthcare

Of course, it is not possible to derive general recommendations from very private experiences, in particular in regard to religious practice. However, what a system of education and healthcare can do is provide a framework that leaves free space and breathing room, thereby counteracting stifling conditions as described above, which can kill creativity, thirst for knowledge, and zest for life. In any case, it seems decisive to allocate time for exploration, rest, and tranquility—to have moments when no specific activity has been scheduled. Moreover, one may alternate between indoor and outdoor activities.

And, very important: instead of putting too much pressure on students or patients, it is better to act like Johannes's father, who appears as an exemplary role model due to his patience and non-directive acceptance of his wife's and son's patterns of self-protection. For many years, the main protagonist of the novel did not want to say a single word about his childhood (Ortheil, 2011, 418). Remaining silent about that which is too painful to be spoken about is a means of regaining control of one's life. This is the reason why many Holocaust survivors and other victims of genocidal violence waited for decades before they, cautiously, recounted their past (see Welz, 2017).

However, we can also learn from Ortheil (2011, 400, 404) that writing can, in fact, have a therapeutic effect in clarifying and structuring one's thoughts and phantasies, in providing fragments of a life story and thus advancing the narrator in his self-transformation and his movement from anxiety to courage, from sadness to joy, from muteness to speech. In a sense, writing was a step on his way to speech. Writing itself is a silent activity; yet, just like speech, it involves words.

More than anything else, the practice of prayer and faith expressed in musical terms, in singing and playing musical instruments, helped the protagonists of the novel to cope with grief grown too large to bear. As Johannes got to know from his uncle, his mother would not be alive anymore without his father. When her fourth child died, it was as if she was about to die as well. The priest who was asked to conduct the funeral tried to remain stoic, but in front of the grave, his eyes welled up with tears, and he could not speak anymore. No one could speak anymore. It was a terrible moment of agony, and no one could see a way out. In this moment, the father of the dead child stepped forward, blew his nose, took a deep breath, and then he prayed in a firm voice: "The Lord is my Shepherd, I lack nothing [. . .]. Even though I walk through the darkest valley, I will fear no evil, for you are with me; your rod and your staff, they comfort me [. . .]" (Psalm 23). Johannes asked his uncle how his father could speak such prayers after the death of four sons. His uncle answered that his father had a deep, unwavering faith that could not be shaken by any event on earth; and thanks to the strength of his faith, a fifth child was born: the narrator of the novel (Ortheil, 2011, 436–38).

Ideally, education results in the development of strong and mature personalities like Johannes' father. However, there is no 'recipe' that could grant the success of this or that didactic method. Neither is there a medical 'cure' that would guarantee the full recovery of heavily traumatized patients. Yet, there are three points we know for sure, which are confirmed by Ortheil's novel:

Firstly, both the educational system and the health system, which are designed to promote human 'flourishing,' should improve on leaving room for and giving time to individual 'growth.' The botanic metaphors may be transferred to human beings to the extent that all living beings have (if I may use this Aristotelian term) an innate *telos* or destination, which consists in fulfilling their own potential: they shall become what they are meant or 'called' to be. While some traits and talents might be genetically co-determined, human freedom implies that our lives are not pre-determined in any fatalistic sense. Rather, we have to respond to the 'call' and find our own ways of living up to the standards implied in it, of growing with the tasks we take upon ourselves, and of unfolding that specific 'seed' which lies within each of us. Yet, just as gardens sometimes need to be cut and cultivated, uncontrolled growth cannot be the aim of institutions responsible for education and healthcare, which is why they also need to incorporate a certain discipline in their regulations, so that they can give direction to individuals searching for their way. However, they cannot and must not prescribe the very content of the call. Therefore, the formation of a 'hearing mind' that listens to the call it has received should be considered integral to education, just as mental healing may include practices of silence which resist the war of words (cf. Muers, 2004, 215).

Secondly, Ortheil's novel demonstrates the importance of shining examples who embody what others are still striving for, and of companions on whom one can place one's trust regardless of whether one makes progress or feels that one has reached an impasse on one's life's journey. As Ortheil has made explicit, trust is key to self-unfolding and interhuman relations that promote the individual's self-expression. While trust may arise 'naturally' as long as it is a child's 'basic trust' in the world, the trust of experienced people can only be preserved if the one(s) trusted prove trustworthy; while trust in the sense of a gift may be received undeservedly, a person's trustworthiness is an ethical achievement (see Grøn & Welz (eds.), 2010; O'Neill 2018). In situations of crisis when mates turn into enemies, sociality is not always the solution or remedy in the case of a loss of trust; after all, the latter destroys the mutuality of the very relations that otherwise would connect us.

How, then, is it possible to flourish despite all odds and under poor conditions, for instance in a refugee camp or in isolation due to COVID-19 quarantines and curfews? In such adverse circumstances, public institutions (closed schools and universities, overcrowded hospitals affected by staff shortage, etc.) can only provide a very limited support. When societal systems have reached their breaking point, we are thrown back to ourselves. At the point where our own resources, too, are about to be exhausted, we need new 'supplies' of mental energy to re-erect our love of life and regard for others. Where can this energy come from, if not (or not exclusively) from our families, friends, teachers, doctors, or other caretakers?

The lesson from Ortheil's novel is—and this is the third point—that in the midst of human tragedy, the individual still has the option to turn towards something or someone transcending the misery in which he or she is entrapped. Johannes and his mother did so by escaping to the little chapel, by praying silently, and by letting themselves be transfigured in the presence of God through the services in Cologne Cathedral. Their spirituality was formed in a Christian context. Representatives of other religions have other ways of encountering the divine that can expand the scope for human imagination and action, or interrupt a routine that has confined the movements not just of the body but also of the mind. In a secularized world, religion is often reduced to privacy, and as it moves out of the public, we risk unlearning age-old cultural practices that have carried many generations before us through all kinds of crises and catastrophes. Hence, Ortheil's novel is a reminder of a treasure that is in danger of being forgotten.

Like plants, persons are drawn towards the light; yet, while sunlight is enough for vegetative growth, the human mind also needs 'light' and 'warmth' in an intellectual and spiritual sense, that is, inspiration and encouragement. However, the crucial moments that open up one's horizons and amplify one's experience cannot be brought about by force; they can only come to pass by grace. For this reason, religious education at schools and spiritual guidance at hospitals should never be imposed upon people who show no interest whatsoever—otherwise one comes to give 'answers' to unasked questions.

3.3 Lightart Sending Signs of Solidarity in Corona Crisis

Let me finally present a work of visual art, a performance in the public space, which not just directs our gazes towards something beautiful, but also includes signs of interhuman solidarity and a reference to the Holy—and thus succeeds in combining aesthetics, ethics, and spirituality.

When houses of worship were closed all over the world in mid-April 2020 in order to maintain distancing measures, messages of hope and unity were projected onto Rio de Janeiro's giant Jesus statue during an Easter Sunday service. With the help of cutting-edge technology, Rio's iconic Art Deco statue "Christ the Redeemer" overlooking the whole city was lit up and illuminated in the national colors of the countries hardest hit by the coronavirus, for instance the blue-white-red of the French flag with the word *espérance,* in order to show solidarity with COVID-19 victims in France and other countries. The words 'hope,' 'thanks,' and 'stay home' became visible in various languages. Furthermore, Christ with his outstretched arms was transformed into a doctor with a lab coat and a stethoscope. Since images of doctors and nurses also intermittently appeared on the figure, this was understood as "a tribute to the healthcare workers on the front line of the pandemic" (Goldstein, 2020).

However, not just the healthcare workers were honored. The light show evoked an additional interpretation, which becomes manifest if it is seen in the context of the Hebrew Bible where God Himself is described as our heavenly doctor: "for I am the Lord, who heals you" (Exodus 15:26). Accordingly, on the photo of the Brazilian archbishop conducting the Easter service, the figure of Christ appears to be hovering in a supernatural purple aura signifying a mystery we cannot grasp but only be touched by.

The contrast to Brazilian president Jair Bolsonaro's messages could not have been more blatant. Bolsonaro told local media outlets that no one would prevent him from coming and going. In an utterly ruthless manner, he jeopardized his own people's health. His selfish attitude was the opposite of what the Czech philosopher Jan Patočka called the "solidarity of the shaken," of those "who are capable of understanding what life and death are all about" (1996, 134). They do so because they have experienced "a strong disturbance of the certainties, big and small, that hold their lives in place"; their "everyday assurances have been overturned" in shock, "which allows them to change their perspective on life" and to regain "the true meaning of their own life through the experience of an actual danger" (Comboni, 2015).

Even if the coronavirus pandemic does not pose a threat to one's own life, it endangers many other people's lives, loved ones near and far—and thus the human community as such. The light show in Brazil invited individuals to give up their egoistic prerogatives in order to be part of a new, unselfish cross-border community that protects all human lives regardless of race, sex, and religion. In portraying Christ as exalted Redeemer-Doctor of humankind and in superimposing the images of healthcare workers, the show managed to symbolize a connection between the human and the divine. Moreover, it universalized the coincidence of professional capability and need for help, which might encourage human beings at the end of their rope to flee to God as a last resort.

Just as the ethical front line of the "solidarity of the shaken" is "quiet, without fanfare or sensation" (Patočka, 1996, 135), although the ruling force might want to destroy the sense of sharing that creates bonds even between strangers, so the religious meaning of redemption is to be sensed in peace and quiet, through listening to the silence of wonder.

As Finn Thorbjørn Hansen rightly remarks, the phenomenon of wonder cannot be controlled or "constructed by pedagogical or philosophical methods" because it is "over and above our wanting and doing" (2011, 167). Wonder 'befalls' us, it 'descends,' so to say—which is why it dislocates us from our expectations and prejudices: we are astonished, as everything appears in a new light (cf. ibid., 170f, with reference to Eugen Fink). Struck by wonder, we become silent and 'listen' to that which unfolds itself in front of our 'inner ears' and begin to 'see' aspects of a situation to which we previously were blind. The state of being 'in' wonder is linked to an attentiveness that differs from our problem-solving modes of being.

'Wonder' in relation to the divine or in a sense of belonging to a place and other people, and not least in rapturing experiences of beauty, is an attitude or state of mind in which one is completely open to the ways in which 'the world' or its 'beyond' begins to 'speak' or disclose itself. Wonder involves the manifestation of something new. In this line, James G. Hart writes: "what is meant by wonder here is that quasi-gracious interruption" of routine (2020, 27). Hart distinguishes between (1) "Aristotelean wonder" of *how* things are, (2) "mystical-theological wonder" *that* things are, and (3) "phenomenological wonder" related to apparition itself, to "the manifestness of first-person experience within which all other wonder emerges" (ibid., 27f). The one who wonders will no longer take for granted what he or she experiences; rather, he or she will suddenly discover something unusual in everyday reality, something strange in the familiar, and be receptive to the unique and puzzling, the marvelous or even miraculous that is encountered in a surprising meeting with 'the ordinary,' which nonetheless seems to contain something 'extraordinary'—as it was the case when the light show appeared in the sky above Rio.[4]

CONCLUSION

We can conclude that a re-humanization of education and healthcare is to be achieved by leading these professions beyond the human, all too human, and its self-absorption. A theological, phenomenological, and hermeneutical, wonder-based approach to our 'being-before-God,' 'being-in-the world,' and 'being-with-others' as the one presented here may also re-direct us to sources of meaning that are not automatically at our disposal, but rather require us to listen to the silence of that which otherwise eludes us, and to open ourselves up for the unpredictable 'visit' of 'the unavailable.'

The latter becomes accessible only to the one who really 'listens' with all senses and responds with heart and soul to the 'call' or 'appeal' inherent in the respective situation, relation, or moment. Exactly because we cannot lay down general rules determining the right way of living for everyone, each of us needs to go on searching for that which is right for him or her. A one-to-one translation of individual responses to other people's specific life situations is impossible, but our common human condition of vulnerability, fragility, and finitude may at least permit a modest transferral of existential insights in how the bonds between us may be strengthened. In the end, human flourishing is not so much an individual project as a communal goal.

Against the backdrop of the current situation, the title of Ortheil's novel, *Erfindung des Lebens,* imposes the question of how we can 'reinvent' life in times of a global pandemic. The present contribution has focused on spiritual, ethical, and aesthetical dimensions of 'wonder' and its life-enhancing effects. As we have seen, it is critical not to cut off religious aspects, although these aspects may be difficult to grasp because they deal with that which transcends our everyday reality and our own limitations. If we are ready to integrate a sober awareness of our own limits into our view of humanity, we are amply rewarded: in outgrowing deadlocked habits, we might surpass ourselves in reaching for a life that remains open to unforeseen marvelousness.[5]

NOTES

1. See ibid.: "In dieser Hypnose begann ich zu beten, aber nicht so, dass ich mir bestimmte Worte ausgedacht hätte, sondern eher, indem ich zunächst zuhörte, wie das Beten in mir von selbst begann."

2. All Bible quotes are cited according to the New International Version (NIV, see https://www.thenivbible.com/).

3. One might ask why sociologist Hartmut Rosa's bestseller *Resonanz* (2016) is not discussed here. The reason is that the main thesis of his book, namely that resonance is the opposite of alienation, leads him to define the latter as a non-responsive

or mute (*stumm*) relation to the world (Rosa 2017, 306). However, this opposition degrades other forms of silence that are not equivalent to muteness, and it excludes negative forms of resonance. For a more detailed critique, see my paper "Listening to Resounding Silence: Post-Traumatic Languages of the Unsayable" (forthcoming). Let me warmly recommend the volume *Attending to Silence: Educators and Philosophers on the Art of Listening* (2012) edited and co-authored by Henny Fiskå Hägg and Aslaug Kristiansen, which gives a more nuanced and multi-faceted account of silence.

4. See photos: https://news.artnet.com/art-world/rio-christ-the-redeemer-doctor-1832199.

5. A warm thank you to my Norwegian colleagues for the truly wonderful research stay at Agder University, Kristiansand, in April 2019, when I became part of the research group preparing this book, and to the team at *Forschungskolleg Humanwissenschaften der Goethe-Universität Frankfurt*, Bad Homburg, where I found the time and leisure for pondering over human flourishing.

BIBLIOGRAPHY

Aristotle, *De anima* (cited according to standard divisions).

Bader, Günter (2016), "Zur Wirklichkeit des Psalters zwischen Patristik und Postmoderne" in: *Og teologi. Festskrift til Carsten Pallesen,* ed. Mads Peter Karlsen and Lars Sandbeck, Copenhagen: Eksistensen, 117–41.

Bar-On, Dan (1989), *Legacy of Silence: Encounters with Children of the Third Reich,* Cambridge, Mass./London, Engl.: Harvard University Press.

Comboni, Isotta (2015), "Charter 77 and the 'solidarity of the shaken'" in: *open democracy,* https://www.opendemocracy.net/en/charter-77-and-solidarity-of-shaken/ (26 March 2015).

Fiskå Hägg, Henny, and Aslaug Kristiansen (2012), "Introduction" to *Attending to Silence: Educators and Philosophers on the Art of Listening,* Kristiansand: Portal Books, 10–14.

Fivush, Robyn (2010), "Speaking silence: The social construction of silence in autobiographical and cultural narratives" in: *Memory* 18:2, special issue: *Silence and Memory*, ed. Monisha Pasupathi and Kate C. McLean, 88–98.

Goldstein, Caroline (2020), "Rio de Janeiro Used Cutting-Edge Technology to Transform Its Giant Jesus Statue Into a Doctor to Honor Healthcare Workers" in: *artnet news,* https://news.artnet.com/art-world/rio-christ-the-redeemer-doctor-1832199 (April 13, 2020).

Grøn, Arne, and Claudia Welz (eds.) (2010), *Trust, Sociality, Selfhood,* Tübingen: Mohr Siebeck.

Hansen, Finn Thorbjørn (2011), "The Phenomenology of Wonder in Higher Education" in: *Erziehung: Phänomenologische Perspektiven,* ed. Malte Brinkmann, Würzburg: Königshausen & Neumann, 161–77.

Hart, James G. (2020), "Some Moments of Wonder Emergent within Transcendental Phenomenological Analyses" in: *Open Theology* 6:1, 27–34, DOI: https://doi.org/10.1515/opth-2020-0004 (January 29, 2021).

Ihde, Don (2007), *Listening and Voice: Phenomenologies of Sound,* 3rd ed., New York: State University of New York Press.

Jørgensen, Dorthe (2004), "Æstetikkens endeligt" in: *Slagmark—Tidsskrift for idéhistorie* 40, 27–40.

Levin, Irene (2013), "The Social Phenomenon of Silence" in: *The Holocaust as Active Memory*, ed. Claudia Lenz, Irene Levin, and Marie Louise Seeberg, Farnham: Ashgate, 187–97.

Morton, Nelle (1985), *The Journey Is Home,* Boston: Beacon Press.

Muers, Rachel (2004), *Keeping God's Silence: Towards a Theological Ethics of Communication*, Malden, MA/Oxford: Blackwell.

O'Neill, Onora (2018), "Linking Trust to Trustworthiness" in: *International Journal of Philosophical Studies* 26:2, 293–300.

Ortheil, Hanns-Josef (2011), *Die Erfindung des Lebens,* München: [Luchterhand Literaturverlag 2009] btb Verlag / Random House.

Patočka, Jan (1996), *Heretical Essays in the Philosophy of History*, Chicago: Open Court.

Risser, James (2019), "Speaking from Silence: On the Intimate Relation Between Silence and Speaking" in: *Journal of Applied Hermeneutics,* 1–14.

Rosa, Hartmut (2017), *Resonanz: Eine Soziologie der Weltbeziehung*, 5th ed., Berlin: Suhrkamp.

Waldenfels, Bernhard (2006), "Das Lautwerden der Stimme" in: *Stimme. Annäherung an ein Phänomen,* ed. Doris Kolesch and Sybille Krämer, Frankfurt am Main: Suhrkamp, 191–210.

Welz, Claudia (2017), "A Voice Crying out from the Wound—with or without Words: On Trauma, Speech, and Silence" in: *Dialog: A Journal of Theology* 56:4, 412–27 (http://rdcu.be/AqxA).

Welz, Claudia (2018), "Self-Knowledge and Self-Deception: Existential Hermeneutics and Psychoanalysis" in: *Hermeneutics and Negativism: Existential Ambiguities of Self-Understanding*, ed. Claudia Welz and René Rosfort, Tübingen: Mohr Siebeck, 237–55.

Welz, Claudia (2019), "A Theological Phenomenology of Listening: God's 'Voice' and 'Silence' after Auschwitz" in: *Religions* 139: 10 (https://www.mdpi.com/2077-1444/10/3/139/pdf).

Chapter 9

Truth-Telling in the Care of the Self

A Path to Serenity and Spirituality in Compressed Times

Randi Edland Kroken

As stated in the introduction to this book, the focus is on how research can contribute to re-enchant and re-humanize health, welfare and education professions to create more space for wondering and openness based on aesthetic, ethical and spiritual dimensions. This aligns with Hermut Rosa's (2020) notion that several practices are out of tune and not resonant to/with human values. Practitioners/professionals need to speak up and fight against these experiences of de-humanization that occur in many modern work places, school systems, welfare systems and health care. However, to speak up and tell the truth about what is going on is not an unproblematic and easy thing to do. Not at all. Therefore this chapter will focus on what it takes to become a 'truth-teller'—a so-called '*parrhesiast*' in ancient Greek—with a special focus on Socrates as the key figure for being a courageous truth-teller. I will show the importance of seeing the conditions and challenges the modern parrhesiast faces when daring to speak up. A parrhesiast today needs to take a humble approach to improve the contexts in which human professionals are enmeshed. Limitations should be taken into account. Inspired by the ideals of ancient Greece and the works on parrhesia by the French philosopher Michel Foucault, I propose that experienced professionals should mentor younger, or less experienced, professionals. Foucault offered an analysis through the lens of Socrates and the ancient Greeks to address contemporary concerns of parrhesia in education.

The word *parrhesia* originates in Greek literature by Euripides (484–407 B.C) and reaches its height of practice during the ancient Greek world of letters from the end of the fifth century A.D. The activity of "free speaking" is characterized by truth, danger, criticism, and duty. The concept "parrhesia" refers to a way of speaking frankly in the sense of "saying everything" that one has in mind (Foucault, 2001, p. 12). It also refers to a relationship between the speaker and what they say as an expression of their own opinion. The expression is not based on rhetoric, but on the speaker's own conviction and subjective belief about what is true. The utterance and the commitment of the parrhesiast are linked to a certain social situation that delineates a difference in status between the speaker and their audience. When the parrhesiast speaks truthfully it creates personal risk and may undermine their professional role culminating in a challenging game between the speaker and their audience.

The parrhesiastes demonstrates courage when expressing oneself in spite of the danger it may entail. A parrhesiastic utterance is connected to two moral qualities. The first is knowing the truth and the second is the necessity to convey such truths to others. This is in contrast to the current trend of remaining "below the radar." Instead of an outer orientation towards external measures Foucault emphasizes that the parrhesiastes first and foremost chooses a specific relationship to himself/herself as a truth-teller rather than being false to oneself:

> If, during a trial, you say something which can be used against you, you may not be using the *parrhesia* in spite the fact that you are sincere, that you believe what you say it is true, and you are endangering yourself in so speaking. For in parrhesia the danger always come from the fact that the said truth is capable of hurting or angering the *interlocutor. Parrhesia* is thus always a "game" between the one who speaks the truth and the interlocutor. (Foucault, 2001, p. 17)

I will focus on the implications of two empirical case studies demonstrating how these experiences derive knowledge from a theoretical concepts. How do such concepts enlighten truth telling in the public sphere within the human professional field today? How can teachers, advisers, and researchers convey knowledge and experience to their students and junior scholars or professionals about truth telling in order to enlighten their entrance in the professional field?

STRUGGLING FOR OTHERS IN PUBLIC SPHERE

The following are two examples of truth-telling practices in the Norwegian welfare system and the personal consequences experienced by these truth-tellers when they spoke up in public domain.

Gains and Losses

Heidi Follett, a social worker, was honored for the best chronicle in 2013 for *The system of stupidity* (*Dumskapens system*). Follett examined how clients in a municipal NAV-supporting system were devalued so that it seemed to demotivate and harm them in various ways (Skårderud, 2020). In the wake of the publication, she was forced to attend a meeting with thirty to forty of her colleagues in front of whom she was blamed for having put them at risk of not being able to fulfill their social contract related to NAV. After the event she was overwhelmed by anxiety and paralyzed by shame. Both the trade union and leadership at work abandoned her and refused communication with her. After taking a week of sick leave she quit her job. When she then applied for support from the NAV-system she was refused admission for eight weeks based on arguments that she had caused the problems herself. Doctors who have treated Follet have documented that she still suffers from Post-traumatic stress disorder (PTSD). When she looks back after seven years she is skeptical of whistleblowing because of the risks one can expect afterwards. She maintains this is particularly true for those with young children.

In the article (Skårderud, 2020) one of Follett's supervisors/managers states that Follett did not foresee, or realize, how her chronicle affected her colleagues and the resulting outcomes. He maintains her colleagues felt suspicious in the wake of her publishing the chronicle.

The following case study demonstrates how truth-telling can result in a process of blaming. The issue at hand appears to vanish and the professionals are thrown into a game they could not anticipate.

THE GREAT SCHOOL PROJECT

In Simon Malkenes's book, *Det store skoleeksperimentet* [*The Great School Project*] (Malkenes, 2018) he describes his experience after publishing a description of the chaotic situation in every-day life within a high school. "The great school project" examines the school of Oslo promoting itself as a school of excellence. The account given by Malkenes contrasted the glorified picture offered by the school. His version of the Norwegian school and educational system reveals a different world than is realized at higher levels, both in the school system itself and at higher political levels. Malkenes had professional experience as a teacher that revealed how daily life in the school created a segregated system that made the pupils ill. Several of the pupils are functionally illiterate. Malkenes's account contrasts with the public's understanding of Norwegian schools described and understood as "the world's best schools," based on the managerial model, with focus on school efficiency and a "test-based accountability" (p. 70) combined with a collaborative management and media training. This managerialism is cultivated as part audit culture and ~~a~~ part ~~of~~ Performance Management branded as in "The Child's Best Interest" (pp. 97, 101).

The publication exploded in the media and Malkenes was blamed for offending the interests of the children. Malkenes argued that the school functioned in a way that led to fatal consequences for vulnerable and weak pupils. The process became personal for Malkenes and after a very turbulent period he went on sick leave. A staff inquiry was opened against him, but subsequently terminated without a formal indictment.[1,2]

Malkenes eventually left Oslo School to work at another school He was honored with Fritt Ord's prize for his brave speech and his active participation in the public sphere. He was honored for being one of the clearest and sharpest voices in debates on developmental traits in Norwegian schools. "The Freedom of Expression Prize" is an acknowledgment accorded to individuals or institutions engaged in activities deemed especially worthwhile in the light of the institution's objects clause.[3] Also the chronicle of Follett was also highly rewarded[4] by an instance at a long distance away from where the play actually occurs. This means that Follett was abandoned in her struggle at a local level, and we shall now look more into what kind of game parrhesia might mean in practice.

TRUTH-TELLING AS A PARRHESIASTIC GAME

The late Foucault (2001) focused on the Parrhesiast as a truth-teller—often translated into English as a kind of "Fearless speech" or "Free speech." In particular he focused on the philosophical parrhesia which first and foremost was represented by Socrates whom Foucault deemed the original parrhesiast (truth-teller). Socrates has become an icon of a Parrhesiast that showed courage. The parrhesia is not a cognitively Cartesian driven subject, but rather driven by the search of truth. Through askèsis and through living a philosophical life (Hadot, 1995; Hansen, 2002), closely connected to a person`s moral character, one builds up a personal courage—a way of purifying oneself. This can lead to a necessity of "self-transformation" in order to gain the truth-access of being oneself. But such demands are a kind of struggle that situate oneself into unanticipated and dangerous situations.

Parrhesia is connected to one`s commitment and an obligation of duty. As said, telling the truth in a way that the interlocuturin might dislike. He might even refuse the truth, which might put the truth-teller at a risk to be exiled or punished, in order to try keep him silent. But a parrhesiastes refuses to obey and continues to speak, because of his feeling of duty to do so. In that way parrhesia is connected both to a freedom and a duty which means that without telling the truth, you are not free.

As a preliminary summary, we can say that free speech is risky and the consequences of expressing oneself freely can be unknown. Looking back on her own experiences Follett realizes how targeted she became when she was confronted with blame from her colleagues. The focus in her chronicle on the relation between the system and the clients turned the gaze on herself as the blamed person. The original issue she raised became moot. Instead she herself became the focus of criticism. Malkenes experienced something similar. From his point of view in the broadcasted program he focused on the effects of a school-system that harmed the pupils. But as the process developed the teacher himself became the problem. We see how the professionals both are exposed to a kind of a transforming process—a kind of a game. Their concerns about the living conditions of their clients are suddenly turned them and they become the objects of criticism rather than the issues they intended to raise.

A closer look at these processes shows how modern truth-tellers becoming players in unforeseen situations. Foucault`s gaze on the parrhesiastic game can enlighten our insight into how the truth might come into play.

ABSORBED IN A NOT FORSEEN GAME

The obligation to tell the truth is seen as a kind of parrhesiastic conduct. Foucault (2001, p. 15) presupposes this as a parrhessiastic play or game. Such a play might lead to consequences that can easily get out of control. Foucault (2001, pp. 36–37) refers to the drama *Ion*, written by the great Greek poet Euripides. This is a game where the story begins with Creusa who became pregnant after a meeting with Apollo. The question was raised whether the pregnancy was a result of a rape or a seduction. Within classical Greek culture seduction was considered a higher criminal offense than rape! A rape was seen as an act without your own will, while seduction was designated an un-faithful act to one's husband or family. When Creusa expected to bear the child, she went to Athens' acropolis. While hiding herself, she gave birth to a son, Ion. Apollo sent his brother, Hermes, who brought up the child in the temple of Delphi. Only Apollo knew Ion's origin. Ion himself didn`t know. Creusa married another man, Xuthus. Since this couple had no children they went to Delphi and asked the oracle if they would have a child. Creusa knows that she had a child with Apollo and she wanted to talk with him, but instead, in the front of the temple they meet Ion. Mother and son are strangers to each other. Apollo concealed the truth. Although the truth was spoken by the gods, they didn`t want to see it. Creusa was still ashamed of what had happened to her, so she pretends that she consulted the oracle on behalf of her friend. Creusa told part of her story to Ion. Ion wanted to fight for truth, while Apollo hid what he knew, so he was an anti-parrhesiastes and a liar, emphasizes Foucault, while Ion and Creusa were the major parrhesiastes.

Although Ion was a true parrhesiastes, brought up in Delphi, he was deprived of the parrhesistic right of free speech in Athens. Despite a mutual parenthood between the cities Sparta and Athens, Ion doesn`t have the right to speak the truth, because of the shift of the place of truth disclosure. In this play there is an explicit shift from the oracular truth at Delphi to Athens. While Apollo had not enough courage to disclose his own faults, he didn`t act as a parrhesiast, but as a liar.

According to Socrates a dialogue might be affected when someone`s pride has been hurt in a way that compels him to recognize claims he was not aware of. This might be perceived as an attack on an interlocutor`s pride, and this might bring the interlocutor to the limits of the parrheisiastic contract in a way that disturbs the way of playing the game. Such a play limits the parrhesiastic agreement. Conquering self-sovereignty is conditioned by a kind of self-examination. Seneca has pointed out the truth emerges from a personal relation which he establishes with himself. However, if the truth is disclosed either by himself or others, that can challenge the self-mastery (Foucault, 2001, p. 165). A general principle is to know thyself. Seneca maintains that self-examination is an ideal, but if one does not succeed in living up to one`s own ambitions, it is especially important to control one`s own anger!

This kind of play has something in common with Gadamer`s approach to how he also sees lived experiences as a play. He defines a play as a mode of being of the work of art itself, not as a kind of an orientation or consciousness. This reflects the approach in *Truth and Method*, where Gadamer (2013) elaborates how we as human beings develop our understanding. "Truth" and "method" are viewed as contradictory concepts. His book is a profound critique of modern scientific thinking, and especially how the human and social sciences have been scientificized. Reality can never be seen as an objective thing we can take for granted. In contrast to former sciences that rejected subjective interpretations and prejudices, is the other way around. Prejudices play a crucial role in the interpretation of new situations so we are able to understand new circumstances.

CHALLENGES IN COMPRESSED TIMES

In this book one of the main reasons for the professionals' unbalanced situation is explained by neoliberalism. NPM, which mainly is driven by neoliberal and economical interests has threatened the vital and crucial values of the professions of health, welfare and education (Hansen, Eide, & Leget, 2023). Although the NPM-movement has been modified by new waves such as new public governance previous ideologies remain influential because they have been internalized in subtle and indirect ways, as a "taken for granted" part of modern leadership and organizational culture and work style. In that sense the values are deep-rooted on a cultural and existential level, not just on the political, management and economic level. As Rosa (2020) emphasizes, the modernization of welfare institutions means that practices are marked by the "shrinking of the present" as a result of an overwhelming acceleration of their lives, which leads to experiences of alienation, existential emptiness and a lack of a meaningful daily life. With the two empirical cases in mind, I will draw attention to some challenges.

A Need of More Knowledge about Daily Professional Practice

Taking the two examples above into account, re-humanizing attempts seems to represent a profound attack on neoliberal values. In social work in particular there is not enough knowledge about daily practice, Jean Gordon's (2018) work reveals that Social Work research shows a surprising lack of research about the day-to-day practice of social work and how lived experiences are affected. She emphasizes the importance of applying narratives and the use of auto-ethnography to support critical best practices, and to strengthen strategies for developing knowledge for practice and professional life. Despite attention which has been offered to practice developments, there is still a need to go more down to earth in the approach to daily practices. Such micro practices of social work and the lived experiences will enrich knowledge about practical circumstances (Gordon, 2018). When we see how a practical and a day-to-day (micro analytic) situation within the human professions impacts relations to clients and then see how this calls for a need to strengthen, re-humanize and support ethical self-care in order to help others.

A Horizontal Splitting: Barries of Conveying Concrete Experiences

A specific dynamic seems to dominate and that procedural responsibility tends to have taken precedence over a concrete moral responsibility (Kroken, 2016 a). There seem to be limits of free speech within, for example, the child welfare system in Norway. When the complexity of child welfare service's work is communicated to leaders and politicians at the management level and in the state child welfare service (Kroken, 2016 a). The concrete responsibility is transformed into an abstract and pragmatic responsibility. Specific children and young people seem to become irrelevant at the «system level». When childcare workers are squeezed it affects their work and within themselves creates a kind of rationalization-process. When practitioners' moral responsibility rationality clashes with an economically and strategically rooted rationality, it leads to a horizontal splitting. While practitioners focus on responsibility for one particular child, the actors at the senior management level rather refer to abstract concepts and talk about the problems in general terms. This represents various rationalities that depicts different worlds of experience (Kroken, 2006; 2016a). Zygmunt Bauman (1997) revealed these mechanisms already in the 1990s when he identified that power was split in a way in which concrete responsibility was abandoned.

Risks of Being Abandoned in a Parrhesiastic Game

The outstanding researcher Marianne Gullestad did not get support from her own colleagues when she published and publicly discussed her research about how dominated the Norwegian discourse was against refugees in Norway. Iver B. Neumanns (2004) shows the difficulties when social anthropologists were challenged to show their ability for parrhesiastic actions. The risk of being abandoned when one act as a parrhesiast became visible. The state of loneliness is reinforced when one is left by colleagues. This shrinks the possibilities for conducting criticism of power (Neumann, 2004, pp. 140–141). It is not what is said that can hinder free speech, but rather the unspeakable processes that become more important than what is verbally expressed (Neumann, 2000, p. 28). These experiences show the fragile effects of being a truth-teller. In Euripides's play Ion we see how Apollo, with his lies, transfers stresses on the other participants in a parrhesiastic game.

A Lack of Meaning When Human Relationships Are Instrumentalized

David Graeber (2019) inquires how daily work is affected by the managerial systems. His interest in this started in informal conversations when he asked people about their work. He discovered people often had huge difficulties conveying what their job really was. These overwhelming stories revealed a lack of meaning in working life and a lack of any feeling of a common purpose. To a large extent these feelings were connected to what Graeber calls 'bullshit jobs.' There is a complex play that seems to be a kind of "strategic ballet" that is poorly linked to solving concrete tasks (Graeber, 2019, p. 186). An expanding bureaucracy creates a kind of ritual delay in a way that leads to a pathological environment where people feel exploited. Merlinda Weinberg & Sara Banks (2019) findings where social workers struggling within what they call the 'unethical climate' of neoliberalism, confirm Graeber`s findings. The increasing managerialism and marketization of welfare services were exacerbated by cuts in welfare provisions following the 2008 financial crisis. They discuss the concepts of 'ethical resistance' and 'ethics work.' They conclude that everyday ethical resistance is not enough to 'make good' in an unethical climate, but they see this as a precursor to social and political resistance. This standpoint seems to have something in common with a philosophical parrhesiast.

FROM A POLITICAL TO A PHILOSOPHICAL PARRHESIAST

Foucault (2001) sees *philosophical parrhesia* as a *new* form of being a parrhesiast. This turning point means a transition from his earlier analyzes of power where, during his last years, he focuses on individual and philosophical life and ethical self-care. This new form has emerged and developed from a political parrhesia. Despite some similarities with the former political parrhesia Foucault characterized this new concept as a "Socratic parrhesia." Belonging to a noble Athenian house was not sufficient. To conquer a prominent position in a city required something more, for example education and more knowledge about how to live a philosophical life. The qualities of the truth telling are tested by the interlocutor`s existence. Socrates philosophical game parrhesia is distinguished from a self-ignorance and the false teaching of the sophists (Foucault, 2001, p. 102). Socrates emphasized the challenge to overcome self-ignorance about one's own situation. Instead of foretelling as the oracle in Athens did, Socrates discourse rather required people to overcome self-ignorance about one`s own situation. Socrates was dedicated to disclosing who you are and your present relation to the truth. The philosopher had to discover and to teach certain truths about the world, and nature, based on an epistemic foundation. This required taking a position to the city, laws etc. Last but not least, parrheisastic activity is endeavoured to celebrate the nature of the relationship between truth and one`s lifestyle, or truth and ethics and aesthetics of the self. This practice tries to shape the specific relations to their own being. Mortality and human values should be rooted in these practices. The overall aim was to change and improve one`s life, but also the lives of others. This new parrhesia implies a complex set of connections between the self and the truth which give access to truth and further knowledge. In light of this the philosophy is seen as a kind of "spiritual guide" (Foucault, 2001, p. 112). Finn Thorbjørn Hansen (2002, 2015) has elaborated how the philosophical parrhesia was derived and developed from the political parrhesia.

THE REQUEST OF BEING ENTITLED TO TELL THE TRUTH

In ancient times slaves were forbidden to speak their mind. If citizens cannot oppose a ruler`s power, they must leave in order to speak up. The person who exercises power is wise only in so far as there exists someone who can use parresia to criticize them, but some limits were put to their power and his command. To do your duty requires that one has positioned oneself against a power instance. The precondition for uttering the truth is that one knows the situation to which the bold expression should be expressed.

An unambiguous precondition was that being a parrhesiast should be based on having a relationship to oneself as a kind of self-love, within oneself. Foucault (2001, p. 143) maintains that any kind of art is derived from truth about yourself which must be learned through *ascesis.* He links this to the concept *mathesis.* Mathesis challenges us to know the certain circumstances we intend to invent. It requires an ability to distinguish a real friend from the more flattering ones! Mathesis is conditioned by a deep understanding of what kind of circumstances one is situated within (Foucault, 2001). To do so one must have a precise understanding of oneself. This is the ultimate precondition of knowing others. This request to *Know thyself* (*gnoti seauton*) (Foucault, 2001, p. 165), which means that we should know our limits for what is possible to achieve. As mentioned, it means expressing the truth that one chooses a lifestyle based on being able to speak frankly against powerful social actors (Foucault, 2001).

Foucault (2001) acknowledges Socrates and Seneca and as main sources for his thinking on parrhesia. One should take a stoic approach to life. Similar to the notion of both Seneca and the parrhesiastic ideal of purifying oneself throughout life, Foucault emphasizes the care of the self as the overall value in this process. Schaanning (2020) believes there is a misunderstanding of the quote "Know yourself." Schaanning says that knowing yourself is, rather, a part of taking care of oneself. These reflections are fruitful in helping us understand the gap between theory and practice that many professionals have been confronted with after finishing their basic education. As we saw, the two professionals strive for fulfilling better conditions for their clients, but they meet several layers of resistance by the public. By going further into what experience means, it might clarify professional preconditions.

As Gadamer points out it is by losing oneself that we are able to grasp the situation. He even emphasizes that the game is superior to the player and absorbs the player. The game is very complex and forms the entire situation and makes the structure of play. This way of seeing experience shows how we might be drawn into an event of truth. In the foreword of the Norwegian edition Espen Schanning (2010, p. 534) expresses it this way: "we simply arrive too late when we want to know what to believe. We are not on solid ground, a lot might happen when we start to experience. We can wonder a lot along the way."

It was first when the professionals in my cases looked back, that they were able to recognize the effects of their own conduct. Seeing it all from a distance opens up more wondering and reflections to the original situation and gives a better space to reflect upon the game they have been involved in. Since newcomers within human professions have quite sparse experience they might lack sufficient understanding. The situation requires that someone more educated and experienced conveys important knowledge to the future professionals.

EDUCATION TO FACILITATE TRUTH-TELLING

Foucault (2001) states if you are exiled, you cannot use parrhesia, and you cannot oppose the ruler`s power. Power limits free speech, and as we saw above parrhesia is not an equally distributed right. Ion was deprived of his right because he was not a citizen of Athens, so the truth remained unsaid. Giving access to mathesis requires education because a parrhesia in and of itself is no longer considered adequate to disclosure the truth, and therefore requires education and personal training. The precise sort of personal training or education needed is also an issue to purify oneself.

Foucault maintains that political, social and institutional concerns about education, which forms the dialogue, are tightly connected to the problem of parrhesia. Education is impacted by the tensions in political field. Foucault emphasizes the importance of receiving the truth from a competent teacher. The crisis regarding *parrhesia* is a problem of truth. It raises a question of who is capable of speaking the truth within the limits of a system where everyone is equally entitled to give their own opinion. This is not entirely a verbal activity, but can rather be an expression for ignorant outspokenness as a result. This represents a problem and a split within itself, and the claim is to take care and ask questions about these relations. History mirrors a certain type of experience, but is also about the silent ones, those at risk to fall out of discussion. Although parrhesia is linked to a personal attitude, as a personal quality and as a virtue useful for the city`s political life, it does not necessarily trigger institutional rights. Hereby one can run a great risk if one criticizes. Without an institutional guarantee, it can be dangerous to talk freely.

According to Gadamer (2013) the profound meaning lies within the experiences itself. When we experience the world we are brought into a kind of play that is impossible to grasp as a whole. He intends to rehabilitate prejudices as conditions of understanding, and he connects this to our way of understanding in practice. In the moment that we`re experiencing a hermeneutic horizon will be raised as a hermeneutic circle. The most basic of all hermeneutic preconditions remains one`s own fore-understanding, which stems from being focused on the same subject. We are challenged to interpret our situation within a polarity of familiarity and strangeness. Such a continuum represents a tension and go into a play between the traditional texts strangeness and familiarity to us (before and present). The true locus of hermeneutic is this *in-between*. Experiencing something new will always expose you to something that might be risky and, in the ultimate consequence, might be dangerous.

Gadamer defines *play* with reference to the "experience of art," and he makes some distinctions:

> . . . this means neither the orientation nor even the state of mind of the creator or this enjoying the work of art, nor the freedom of subjectivity engaged in play, but the mode of being of the work of art itself. In analyzing aesthetic consciousness we recognized that conceiving aesthetic consciousness as something that confronts an object does not do justice to the real situation. This is why the concept of play is important in my exposition. (Gadamer, 2013, p. 106)

Even if the players themselves know that play is only a game and often defined it as a purpose, they still are not capable of knowing the whole situation. Understanding is always for the time being. To experience the real world might mean that one exist in a not knowing position. Ion becomes quite helpless under new circumstances in Athens. The situation of the two professionals have some similarities while their utterances harms their former interlocutors and their aims are quite opposite. While their employers are dedicated to maintain a positive reputation, the professionals rather want to convey the truth they experience in their local surroundings. These two opposite horizons seem to fall apart, and they can be seen as two split horizons. Gadamers (2013) underlines the importance of being aware of traditions, prejudices and preconception. However, for those new to the professional field, they might not have sufficient knowledge of circumstances. As seen above, the two truth-tellers were both thrown into a game that was nearly impossible to understand in scope and complexity. Teachers and the more experienced professionals can convey knowledge about power relations within the field, in order to prepare young students to handle the dilemmas within potential situations. Without realistic preparation, one might freeze and be unable to act.

THE CARE OF THE SELF IN ORDER TO CARE FOR OTHERS

Gadamer's view of experience leads in an appropriate way to Foucault`s lectures about *The hermeneutics of the subject* in 1981–1982. Here he gives more space for the care for the self in order to subsequently (in the) care for others. Now it becomes a question of caring of oneself, for the sake of oneself. Hadot (1995, in Hansen, 2002) has elaborated Foucault's concept of ethical self-care, and the care for others, society, nature, etc. He sees ethical self-care as a life-aesthetic creation process. Foucault understands life as a work of art, where the individual, as an artist, must step aside so that the art itself can be expressed in order to transcend an unambiguously subjective aesthetic feeling or construction.

But how can one understand the logic of the situations within the human professions field? We shall move a step forward to understand how truth-tellers are affected in our time. Just before his death, Foucault completed volumes two and three of the history of sexuality. In his former research he analyzed how subjects are constituted through discursive techniques (knowledge) and dominance techniques (power). The focus is now more on how we shape ourselves through "the techniques of the self." This subjectivation appears to be an active process, but taking the step into practice and applying the techniques is still not a free choice. It meant a turn towards attention to ourselves and thus a connection to a self-creation. Foucault`s two volumes on the history of sexuality deal with various forms of control and management of one's own behavior. These are "self-relationship technologies" or "self-relationship practices"—a kind of self-cultivation from the 300s BC to 200 AC. The philosophical turn in Foucault`s development does not mean that he rejects the critical philosophical perspectives on science in his earlier thinking, but he has shifted from a focus on the history of science, and started to examine the problematizations of ancient times with increased focus on morality. There is still talk of examining how areas of knowledge are constituted by virtue of a number of practices. However, now it is not about science, but rather, he examines strategies and practices that enable and stage certain forms of morality. The decisive factor is how individuals work with themselves in order to constitute themselves as sexual or a moral subjects in the deepest sense. Care for the self is understood as the care of one's own self. (Schaanning, 2020, p. 284).

Foucault's gaze on new parrhestic practices showed that the political vocabulary was not sufficient. The subject itself is obliged to tell the truth and to be true to what one`s experiences. This philosophy takes into account a kind of existential, and also a spiritual and esthetic kind of self-care, as a guidance in life. In total, this represents a practicing philosophy which, in the deepest sense, means a choice of a life style focused on the aesthetic and existential practice described as "Ethical Self-Care" (Hansen, 2015).

I think it is of crucial importance to take into account the insight of Gadamer, who emphasizes that *all* experience is understood in principle as a confrontation with something insecure, even with nothingness.[5,6] In the Norwegian translation of Gadamer's *Truth and Method* it is translated in a bit more moderate way:

> . . . experience is initially always experience of negation: something is not what we supposed it to be. In view of the experience that we have of another object, both things change-our knowledge and its objects. We know better now, and that means that the object itself "does not pass the test." The new object contains the truth about the old one. (Gadamer, 2013, p. 363)

Although I have claimed that one can enlighten the situation of young idealistic professionals by educating them (in advance), one must admit that when it comes to the concrete experiences you will in principle never know what you are going be exposed to. The more the world is divided, the more difficult it might be to know what you can expect. Given the fact that modern welfare organizations are often split into different worlds, the more we need to know that we can understand the underlying mechanisms. This kind of splitting can be understood as a consequence in the wake of a neo-liberalistic governing. Dany-Robert Dufour (2008, in Madsen, 2011) describes these processes as a kind of schizophrenic mechanisms. He sees this as a contrast to reactions in former times, reactions that were more reminiscent of neurotic conduct. Although this is not meant as absolute diagnosis, it refers to an overall conduct pattern—a kind of an inner splitting, which means that Freud's neurotic subject is weakened, and an inner sense of guilt is diminished. The ambitions we saw in the two stories showed how the publicly painted picture differed from the inner experiences. Revealing the inner experiences destroys the public impression, and in that way the utterances of the professionals destroy or harm the reputation of the school or the welfare institution as a system. This process has resulted in a polarization and a splitting characterized as either black or white.

We cannot take the world and reality for granted, but have to go into it, inquire and find out. In this way, our starting point is a "not knowing position." In Foucault`s focus on the "the aesthetics of existence," he challenged humans to look upon life as a work of art. This can be seen as an irresponsible attitude if it is not based on the commitment of humans. On the other hand, it can be seen as an expression of the "will to form" intimate associations with being able to live life ethically, as a type of life art. However, this requires handling dilemmas in a dynamic way.

The use of networks plays a prominent role in modern organizations. The request is to achieve effective relationships through networking that can be mutually fruitful. But the risk is to ignore awareness of what is true and trustful. The temptation might lead to a kind of instrumental use of each other in order to achieve benefits for ourselves. "Then the welfare of the other is not seen as unique and valuable in itself, but rather as a goal to achieve our own benefits. Or rather, "The other person in the relationship can be a subject as long as the person serves my own interests," says Hilde Nafstad, Rolv Blakar and Rand-Henriksen (2009, p. 158).

Arne Johan Vetlesen (2020, p. 144), has explored Foucault`s relationship to neoliberalism. He found that the relationship between "governors and governed" are not sufficiently examined. He asks if Foucault`s criticism of the relation between the state and its institutions, such as schools, prisons and hospitals, undermined the legitimacy of the welfare state when it was attached to new right-wings. Vetlesen maintains that freedom can only exist in interaction with security. This is also the case in the professional field, as expressed s in this quote, formulated by Rønnestad and Skovholt (2011, p. 56): "the security-insecurity paradox." Only when one is safe and secure, one can open up to feel insecure.

THE CARE FOR THE SELF IN PARRHESIA

It was first with the distance of retrospection that the professionals saw the depth in their own experiences. Simon Malkenes expresses his sorrow thinking back on his obligations for his pupils:

> I have taken part every year in the graduation and after that I have seen my students walk the road to the metro with diplomas in their hands. I am thinking that it is most beautiful being a teacher, to see the students go out into the world, on their way in life. . . . After the event some students come solemnly to say goodbye. Some give a shy hug. Others take a serious farewell and they say "Thank you" (. . .). Together with good colleagues, I stood with a lump in my throat and a thumping teacher's heart and watched them go. But not this time. (Malkenes, 2018, p. 286)

His heartfelt grief is palpable, at the same time as he feels great gratitude for having been able to experience the beautiful fellowship with his students, he also feels a humble feeling towards the pupils who have given him so much. This moment is closely linked to the experience of what is true and something that is resonant with the inner feeling of being human. I think in this case we are dealing with what Foucault calls "parrhesia in the care of the self." Being resonant with this type of experience has something to do with being committed to one's own experience of truth.

I think also the worries about being a whistleblower that Heidi Follett (Skårderud, 2020) expresses when she is looking back on her experiences is also a sign of how deeply such activities affect the professional in a personal way. Follett is concerned that internal cultures in general seem to prevent free speech, and she sees a challenge that someone can use their voice to convey the effects of negative mechanisms of a saturated streamlining public sector.

We see how standing up and speaking freely represent an important dimension of taking self-care, despite worries and pains. Still, the knowledge from Foucault and ancient times points to some reservations which are related to shrinking possibilities to do so. This matter underlines the importance of giving more attention to the care of the Self. And we see how the situations spontaneously call for attention in the same moment (not as a more cognitively oriented reaction suggested by Habermas). An ethical approach is to a high degree linked to a lasting commitment to values in your own life and not a superficial orientation, in the meaning of Kierkegaard`s conceptualization of the word "aesthetic" (Kroken, 2016 b). The experiences sound to be a very deep-rooted, existential ones that correspond to what Hansen (2023, p. 31) calls an "ontological homecoming." Such experiences can give access to the sort of life that calls for more silence and that brings us into a more humble space so that we attain a spiritual inner freedom, and enter into a kind of a spiritual wonder (Hansen, 2023).

Wineberg and Banks (2019) warn against standing alone. This kind of approach has something in common with Foucault's concept of the political parrhesia. Although these researchers' underlining of a collective support is crucial, I will ask if it is a sufficient approach. According to Seneca it is crucial to defend and strengthen one's own personal relation to truth. This requires that one has trained oneself to handle such tensions and challenges—the self-mastery of the person him/herself /thyself. Seneca challenges self-examination and the ability to control one`s own anger! The complexity of games challenge the importance of listening to one's own experiences. Taking into account Gadamer's concept of negation, we are not able to know in advance what is going to happen to us. But our prejudice might still strengthen the truth teller's hermeneutic truth experience, despite uncertainty. Foucault (2001) emphasizes that all experiences are particular. The necessity is always to inquire the specific context as such!

The huge gap and the split horizons above, makes it worth thinking about the standpoint of Svend Brinkmann (2016) when he reminds us of the art of limitation. There seems to be a general notion that one in a modern democratic society is free to criticize. The examples in this chapter have shown the opposite. Brinkman emphasizes that a boundless notion of freedom can be rather paralyzing. He refers to Foucault's "the aesthetics of existence" in order to look upon life as a work of art. Especially when we know how dangerous truth telling might be, we should take into account the ability to tell the truth under certain circumstances. Brinkmann calls for a need to limit the rules, so that not only the strongest will win (Brinkmann, 2016, p. 118).

This book opens up the meaning of wonder as a phenomenon beyond language. Being in the open and in a not-knowing position can strengthen our caring as an active listener. Being in touch with life phenomena can offer human professionals a lifelong-learning process and build a stronger intuition to know and the courage to act later. As we saw above, even brief moments can give unexpected experiences and appear as a gift, as grace and open a space for human flourishing and spirituality, as we saw in the authentic moment above (see Hansen, 2023). Being in wonder as a cognitive and ethical experience can strengthen the ability to handle, or at least understand, a situation better than if one just takes the expected situation for granted. Without taking into account various outcomes, one might be thrown into danger. The meaning of being open and acknowledging the uncertainty in a situation is crucial. The less wonder, the more fragile an outcome might become (Hansen, Eide, & Leget, 2023).

CONCLUSION

A complex game exposed how truth-telling can come into play. The huge challenge is to find out more about how truth-telling affects human professions today. We need to look more deeply into what room there is for expanding and re-humanization by strengthening ethical self-care practices. At the same time there is undoubtedly a certain possibility in expanding the space with more awareness of limits and what lies in "know thyself" (and others). Leget (2021) focuses on the importance of evolving an inner space. I think it is especially crucial to see the relationship between meaning and connectedness on various levels: personal, interpersonal and institutional. Leget warns against using spiritual care as an instrument in order to help clients in dealing with their situation. Rather, he recommends an alternative, alias Rosa`s approach to the existential dimension, for instance by focussing more on the respect for otherness than psychological perspectives often seem to do.

From the ancient times there was a claim that called for a need for being educated. Truth-telling is a quite complex play, requiring that truth-tellers (especially students) should receive the truth from more competent teachers. As Gadamer has shown, experience in principle means a confrontation with negation.

The recognition of this fundamental understanding shows the importance of strengthening existential, philosophical, aesthetic, and spiritual self-care. Hansen (2023) shows the importance of strengthening the ethical self-care practices. Such an approach opens up the possibility for experiencing wonderful things in life. Hansen underlines that the greatest teacher in ethical self-care is not ourselves, but wonderful things that we can learn from and learn through taking part in ethical self-practices. Foucault`s quote in the beginning of this chapter challenges us to realize the activity of truth-telling, and to realize how the truth-teller is dependent on the relation to power!

NOTES

1. https://www.nrk.no/osloogviken/ingen-personalsak-mot-malkenes-1.14022553. NRK 25.4.18. Downloaded 1.4.20.

2. https://www.vg.no/nyheter/innenriks/i/9mVwbp/oslos-skoledirektoer-avslutter-personalsak-mot-simon-malkenes. VG 24.4.18. Downloaded 1.4.20.

3. http://www.frittord.no/en/priser/fritt-ords-pris/. Downloaded 1. 4. 20.

4. NRK Ytrings kronikkonkurranse: Makt/avmakt (https://www.nrk.no/kultur/kritiserer-nav-systemet-fra-innsida-1.10997596). Downloaded 1.4.20.

5. and even named as the meeting with "the nothingness." In Norwegian: "Erfaring er (. . .) I virkeligheten alltid en erfaring av intetheten. Det er ikke slik vi trodde" (Gadamer, 2010, p. 395).

6. In the original edition, Gadamer (2010, p. 363) says it this way: Erfahrung is also Erfahrung des menschlichen Endlichkeit. Erfahrung im eigentlichen Sinne ist, wer ihrer inne is, wer weiss, dass er der Zeit und der Zukunft nicht Herr ist.

REFERENCES

Bauman, Z. 1997. *Moderniteten og Holocaust,* Vidar-forlaget A/S, Oslo.

Brinkmann, S. (2018). *Gå glipp: om begrensningens kunst i en grenseløs tid.* Oslo: Press.

Dufour, D. R. (2008). *The Art of Shrinking Heads: On the New Servitude of the Liberated in the Age of Total Capitalism.* Cambridge: Polity Press (NB-Shrinking).

Foucault, M. (1983; 2001). *Fearless Speech* (red. Joseph Pearson). New York, NY: Semiotext(e).

Gadamer. H. G. (2010). Hermeneutik I. Wahrheit und Methode. Grundzüge einer philosophischen Hermeneutik. Tübingen: Mohr Siebeck Tübingen (7. Auflage).

Gadamer. H. G. (2010). *Sannhet og metode*—grunntrekk i en filosofisk hermeneutikk. Oslo: Pax.

Gadamer, H. G. (2013) *Truth and Method.* London: Bloomsbury Academic.

Graeber, D. (2019). *Bullshitjobs.* UK/USA/Canada/Ireland/Australia/India/New Zealand /South Africa: Penguin Books.

Gordon, J. (2018). The Voice of the Social Worker: A Narrative Literature Review. *British Journal of Social Work.* 48, 1333–50.

Hadot, P. (1995). *Philosophy as a Way of Life. Spiritual Exercises from Socrates to Foucault.* Oxford: Blackwell.

Hansen, F. T. (2002). *Det filosofiske liv—et dannelsesideal for eksistenspædagogikken.* Kbh.: Gyldendal. (Phd-afhandling).

Hansen, F. T. (2015). The Philosophical Practitioner as a Co-Researcher. In Fatic, A. and Amir, L. *Practicing Philosophy.* Cambridge: Cambridge Scholars Publishing.

Hansen, F. T. (2023). Apophatic and existential wonder as a humanizing force In Hansen, F. T., Eide, S. B., Leget, C. (Ed.) *Wonder, Silence and Spaces for Human Flourishing. Towards a humanization of the professions of Health & Care, Welfare and Education,* New York, Lexington Books, pp. 21–45.

Hansen, F. T., Eide, S. B., Leget, C. (2023). Introduction Chapter. In Hansen, F. T., Eide, S. B., Leget, C (Ed.) *Wonder, Silence and Spaces for Human Flourishing. Towards a humanization of the professions of Health & Care, Welfare and Education,* pp. 21–45. New York, Lexington Books.

Kroken, R. (2016a). Vilkår for maktkritikk I Kroken, R og Madsen, O.J. (red.) *Forvaltning av makt og moral i velferdsstaten—fra sosialt arbeid til arbeid med deg selv* Oslo: Gyldendal, ss. 64–85. ISBN: 978–82–05–49269–1.

Kroken, R. (2016b). Mellom etikk og estetikk. Utfordringer i sosialt arbeid I Trysnes I. og Eide, S. B. (red.). *Sosionomutdanning på Sørlandet. Festskrift ved 25 års jubileet høsten 2016.* Kristiansand: Portal Forlag, ss. 33–47. ISBN: 978–82–8314–103-0.

Madsen, O. J. (2011). Nyliberalismens sosialpsykologi; Dany-Robert Dufours kritikk av nyliberalismen. *Agora,* Vol 29, nr. 1, pp. 94–117. ISSN: 0800–7136.

Malkenes, S. (2018). *Det store skoleeksperimentet: makt, barn og forretningshemmeligheter i «verdens beste skole».* Oslo: Manifest. 379.4821 (NB)379.1,373.12, 373.238, 379.481.

Nafstad, H., Blakar, R., Rand-Henriksen, K. (2009). Individualisme og fellesskapsverdier i dagens norske samfunn. I Nafstad og Blakar (red.). Fellesskap og individualisme. Oslo: Gyldendal akademisk.

Neumann, I. B. (2002). Forord I Foucault, M. *Forelesninger om regjering og styringskunst*. (ss. 7–38). Oslo: Cappelen akademisk.

Neumann, I. B. (2004). Maktkritikk som antropologiens adelsmerke. Norsk antropologisk tidsskrift 15(3), 133–44.

Rosa, H. (2020). *Resonance. A Sociology of our relationship to the world.* Cambridge: Polity Press.

Rønnestad, Michael Helge & Skovholt, Thomas M. (2011). Om terapeuters profesjonelle utvikling og psykoterapiveileding i et utviklingsperspektiv, I: Michael Helge Rønnestad & Sissel Reichelt (red.), Veiledning i psykoterapeutisk arbeid. Universitetsforlaget. ISBN 978–82–15–01756–3. pp. 45–66.

Schaanning, E. (2010), Forord. I Gadamer. H. G. (2010). *Sannhet og metode—* grunntrekk i en filosofisk hermeneutikk. Oslo: Pax.

Schaanning, E. (2020). *Omsorgen for seg selv.* Oslo: Pax Forlag.

Skårderud, J. R. (2020). Betaler dyrt for å si fra. *Klassekampen,* 1. juli 2020, pp. 10–11.

Vetlesen, A. J. (2020). Foucault om nyliberalismens idèhistorie. *Agora* (38), nr.3–4, pp. 120–55.

Weinberg, M. & Banks, S. (2019). Practising Ethically in Unethical Times: Everyday Resistance in Social Work. *ETHICS AND SOCIAL WELFARE.* https://doi.org/10.1080/17496535.2019.1597141. ISSN: 1749–6535 (Print) 1749–6543 (Online) Journal homepage: https://www.tandfonline.com/loi/resw20.

A Postscript

From Theoretical Reflections to Humanizing Practices

Carlo Leget and Finn Thorbjørn Hansen

In the introduction of this book, we introduced the phenomenon of beautiful moments in nursing: moments that are normally seen as an exception, not to be taken seriously. These moments of wonder are characterized by a strong sense of meaningfulness and 'humanity,' that seems to escape or transcend what can be grasped in the dominant language of science and professionalism. These moments become ineffable when wanting to document and measure them by evidence-based scientific methods. And yet it is the call of, and the call in, those moments that reconnects us with the meaningfulness and importance of caring and engaging in human relations.

In this book we have explored moments and dimensions like these, which are not lived to their full potential because they fall outside of the control mode we are used to in our professional lives. All the authors of this collection of essays have shown—each in their own way and using different theoretical perspectives—the potential and promise of wonder, silence and spaces for a re-humanization of professions in health care, welfare and education. At the end of this collection of essays we will reflect on the question how the insights of this book might challenge the human professions as we know them. We see the following steps or tasks that all contribute to the same project, but focus on different audiences and professions:

1. promoting a language to give words to these experiences of wonder and human care;

2. bringing the epistemological foundation of our approach in dialogue with the mainstream approach of evidence-based knowledge and science;
3. introducing the insights of our approach into the education of professionals in health care, welfare and education;
4. developing ways to implement our approach to the various practices of healthcare, welfare and education.

FINDING WORDS FOR THE INEFFABLE

A first task that we see for the further humanization of professions in health care, welfare and education is to develop a language to give words to these experiences of beauty, wonder and human caring. How do we create spaces and an awareness of the importance of these moments in human science and human-centered professional work, so they can be recognized, and can be seen as important heuristic experiences that are "food for thought"?

Although language has the risk of 'killing' the richness of wonderment by putting it in terms of what we already know, at the same time language is a prerequisite of being able to communicate about something. We need language that is evocative and open enough to mobilize people, and helps them to become in resonance with their humanizing intuitions and moments. Here the arts are helpful.

In the chapter written by Merel Visse, Aslaug Kristensen, and Claudia Welz we sense how by relating to and dwelling from within lived experiences art, poetry and novels can open a region of intuitions and visions, that our rational, systematic, discursive and method-driven scientific languages are not able to sense and grasp. "Your Thoughts Don't Have Words Every Day," as the poet Emily Dickinson expresses it, catches eloquently what is at stake in moments of deep inspiration or contemplations. Words will always be the result of an impression, an intimation, that seeks an expression. Can we think and wonder without words? Is wonder, or the spark of artistic inspiration, coming from a saturated silence, a silence that is filled with an excess of meaningfulness that wants to be expressed by the human? Why is it that art, say a poem—and even thoughtful poetics, that is, written contemplations made by a poet reflecting on the praxis from within her living experiences of writing poems—can express much better than a scientific report or clear logical definition or group concept mapping, what is at stake in human affairs of caring and human flourishing?

We think that human science and qualitative research need a sensitivity, receptivity and reflexivity towards these ineffable experiences or living mysteries in our everyday lives. In the experience of art—and in the experience of philosophizing—we encounter an opening to and reception of a 'truth experience' that transcends the analytical 'logical-truth' and 'empirical-knowledge' verified by the methodological means proper to nature and social science. Or as Hans-Georg Gadamer states: "Hence, together with the experience of philosophy, the experience of art is the most insistent admonition to scientific consciousness to acknowledge its own limits"(Gadamer, 2006, pp. xxi-xxii).

In this book we have in various ways pointed to different forms of wonder-based 'slow thinking' inspired by research disciplines such as existential and ethical phenomenology, art-based research approaches and through a discourse-critical approach that include so-called "Ethical Care of the Self."

SEEKING A DIALOGUE ABOUT EPISTEMOLOGY

This brings us to the second task. We need to start a dialogue about the epistemological underpinnings of the mainstream approaches in the natural sciences and the social sciences searching for evidence and proofs. After many centuries, the medieval ideal of a place in society where the best of all available ('universitas') knowledge would be gathered and brought to a higher level, has resulted in an academic institution in which different paradigms exist next to each other: the positivist paradigm of natural and medical sciences; the social-constructivist paradigm of the social sciences; and the phenomenological-hermeneutic paradigm of the humanities.

One problem is that academics working in one of these traditions hardly speak or publish with each other, for the endless specialization and endless production of often competitive knowledge production has resulted in different silo's existing next to each other rather than an academic community being in conversation with each other.

A second problem deeply rooted in the minds of many people is a supposed hierarchy between the three paradigms, placing the positivist paradigm at the top scientific knowledge and the phenomenological-hermeneutic paradigm at the bottom. Scientific knowledge is supposed to be acquired according to the methods developed by the natural sciences: a point of view that leaves only space to other paradigms at the price of being seen as less scientific.

As Gadamer has convincingly shown in his philosophical landmark book 'Truth and Method,' however, it is impossible to develop a method for the humanities (*Geisteswissenschaften*) parallel to the natural sciences. The reason for this is that any such attempt would fail to understand what the main task of the humanities is (understanding networks of meaning versus explaining causal relations) and how the human mind works when interpreting the artifacts and texts of human beings (being discursive and based on an increased capacity of understanding through *Bildung*).

A dialogue on epistemology is difficult to achieve, however, for a number of reasons. A first difficulty is a cultural one. Western culture focuses on utilitarian principles like the maximation of pleasure and the avoidance of pain. The standard of living that is connected with pleasure is characterized by a materialist and consumerist approach to life. The natural sciences are at the basis of an impressive technological revolution that has increased the life standard in the West (at the cost of exploiting both nature and people living in other parts of the world) and are considered to be the most important and stable guarantee for that life standard. All this is secured by a neoliberalist mind-set according to which in the end everything is defined, understood and assessed according to an economic rationality. And again, the natural sciences play a pivotal role in providing the evidence bases for economy as a science.

Because natural sciences are seen as the most secure basis for economic prosperity and a high standard of living, their position is hard to challenge. Still there are serious reasons to argue for a more equal treatment of different paradigms of knowledge. In the first place, it is becoming more and more obvious that an unlimited economic growth based on the exploitation of people and nature leads to unprecedented catastrophes like the most recent climate crises and humanitarian disasters caused by the growing divide between the rich and the poor in this world. Secondly, social scientists like Hartmut Rosa (2016, 2019) have shown that the neoliberal society in the end eats its own children by a logic of acceleration that consumes citizens who are reduced to work forces, and does not deliver the happiness it promises, because it can only sell promises of happiness, instead of happiness itself. The reason for this is that valuable human experiences are based on what he calls 'resonance,' which can neither be controlled nor produced.

In a culture that understands science as positivist science and has made people believe this kind of knowledge is at the basis of prosperity and happiness, it is hard to make a case for a more balance between different academic knowledge traditions. It is as if Maslow's pyramid decides here between what cannot be missed as a basis of human existence, and what are nice-to-haves on top of this basic level of prosperity. Changing the mindset of a culture is a huge challenge that will require different conversations with different stakeholders. As regards the conversation between scientists in academia, this discussion has to be a philosophical one, challenging academics to reflect on their own values in life and their responsibility in upholding an economic system that is ethically no longer defensible.

A NEED FOR CHANGE IN PROFESSIONAL EDUCATION

A third task is to develop ways to implement the insights of our approach into the education of professionals in health care, welfare and education. In many countries there are initiatives that are helping to open up to these dimensions, like bioethics, and more recently: narrative based medicine and medical humanities. Initiatives like these are important and need to be developed further. When young professionals are introduced into wonder based inquiries next to their natural science based approaches, they will learn to speak a second language bringing them in resonance with their humanity.

But there is a second, more radical change in professional education that can be developed, based on the different and complementary forms of knowledge that have been described in this book. Professional education in health care, welfare and education is based on both the positivist and the social-constructivist paradigms, training young professionals in utilitarian, pragmatic and problem solving modes of knowledge. In the best cases there are elements of the phenomenological-hermeneutic paradigm of the humanities. We ask: Do we also need what the American philosopher William Franke (2020) has termed an "Apophatic Turn" in critical thinking, that is, a turn that goes beyond the linguistic and pragmatic turn, which was so well-known to and used by theorists and human scientists of the late twentieth century? This turn, Franke claims, will give space to an acknowledgment of the importance of "non-knowing" as a gateway into deeper contemplative understanding not only of human affaires but also 'more-than-human' events and phenomena. Do we need—inspired by the artists and their unique experiences and practices—a shift from talking about research theory to 'research poetics' in order better to get in resonance and dialogue with "die Sache Selbst," that is, the living phenomenon as a mystery that 'talks back' to us? We think so. This book has been an attempt to point in that direction.

MAKING IT WORK IN PRACTICE

A fourth task is developing ways to implement our wonder-based or apophatic approaches to the various practices of health care, welfare, and education. In Denmark, Wonder Labs have been developed in different forms in hospices, hospitals, design and welfare education, and in innovative departments of public organizations adapted to the possibilities and potential of the people working in different practices. These Wonder Labs are transformative and make use of new modes of knowledge, or rather inspired 'non-knowing,' to be integrated in professional practices (Hansen, 2015, 2016, 2018; Hansen & Jørgensen, 2020, 2021).

The Wonder Lab is just one practical example of how to develop a nuanced understanding of ways to get in 'resonance' with the world, as Harmut Rosa urges us to do. And by its emphasis on cultivating dialogical spaces for the sense of wonder, the Wonder Lab also paves the way to a receptivity towards the living mysteries (Marcel, 1950) or the spontaneous and meaning-giving life phenomena, which the Danish philosopher K.E. Løgstrup has made us aware of as ethical callings in the midst of our everyday lives.

The five momentums in the Wonder Lab are illustrative for the kind of practices in education and professional training that this kind of wonder-based and apophatic thinking demands. In the first phenomenological momentum the participants notice that "something calls," something is resonating with them in a lived experience. The second hermeneutic momentum helps the participants to ask and reflect upon "What do we hear in this resonance? How do we comprehend this resonance? What does this resonance want us to become attentive to?" The third momentum is connected to an expansion of the current knowledge and value horizons of the participants when listening to how this "lived resonance" also seems to be resonating with the Grand Narrative of Wisdom that art, philosophy, and theology through the history of humanity have provided us with. The fourth existential momentum encourages the participants to dwell upon the question: "How do I resonate with what is calling? How do I live and experience this resonance in my own life?" And finally, the fifth 'momentum of phronesis' in the Wonder Lab asks the participants to collectively reflect upon the insights and practical wisdom that they have gained through this Bildung process. "What are we concretely called to do right now? What practical changes and first steps would be optional and wise to do now in order to change the current order and ways of living, working, and organizing?"

These are examples of momentums and questions that we believe professionals and students in healthcare, education, and welfare would benefit from when wanting to re-humanize their practices and cultivate their senses of the ineffable and unattainable and unavailable meaning-giving life phenomena. Of course, many other forms of artistic, spiritual, playful, philosophical, and creative practices and methods can be pointed to here in order to enhance such a sense for wonder and the ineffable in life. Our main point is only to encourage a development of a myriad of educational and professional practices that can keep our senses of the enigmatic and mystery open in the midst of our work and life per se.

In other words, the insights developed in this book can begin to bear fruit only when they are implemented in practices of health care, welfare, and education. We could also put it this way: their transformative humanizing power can only begin to work once they have become a part of daily practices. Transforming these practices is a process, in which the people taking part in a practice and the way in which they work together are transformed simultaneously. The transformation of professionals already starts in the professional education discussed above. But it can only be successful when practices are structured in such a way that there is space for this dimension, and when this dimension is present in the way professionals are doing their work.

In the past decades a similar (and related) effort in a humanizing direction has been done in the field of ethics. At this moment, e.g., most health care institutions have an ethical board and in many countries there are ethical case deliberations. These are structural examples of how an institution can promote attention for the ethical dimension of their work. But as such they are not a guarantee that this ethical dimension is secured. An ethical board can become a bureaucratic and authoritarian institution in itself, that specializes in gate keeping and avoiding risks; and ethical case deliberations can become places where power struggles flourish because an unsafe atmosphere hampers an honest exchange between participants from different professions (Kohlen, 2009). For the implementation and flourishing of the ethical dimension something more is needed: a transformation of the way professionals work and are aware of this dimension in their daily work. And this can only be realized in a safe atmosphere, that invites people to share their vulnerability and train their receptiveness.

Creating spaces for the transforming power of silence and wonder in relation to human centered professions is not a new phenomenon in the North-Atlantic world. Perhaps this book is rather a rediscovery of a tradition that has been alive in the past two hundred years where religious congregations took care of the care for the sick and the education of children. Looking at these practices from a secular perspective, it is interesting to observe that time and space were structured in a way that enabled to constantly open up to the dimension of thankfulness and wonder: during the day there were different moments of contemplation and prayer, and the buildings were decorated with different pieces of religious art, inviting to connect one's own story with the stories of a particular religious traditions. This book has no restorative intentions, but it is clear that we can learn from practices that have been effective for many centuries.

One of the challenges one faces when trying to create spaces of silence and wonder is to make room for a different mindset than the task-oriented efficiency mode most professionals have becoming used to. That means that one has to invite people to enter a defined space with different rules as a laboratory to experiment with silence and wonder. The wonder labs are an interesting example of such a transformative space.

A PERSPECTIVE BEYOND HUMANIZATION

During the years of writing this book, the world has changed in a way only few experts would have imagined and predicted. The Covid 19-pandemic has laid bare many problems related to the way Western societies have been organized, and a widespread awareness has grown that many of these problems find a common ground in an anthropocentric worldview that overlooks the entanglement of human beings with nature. What does this mean for the striving for humanization as developed in this book? Are the contributions in this volume to humanizing education, welfare, and health care a step back towards an anthropocentrism that should be abolished to the favor of a paradigm decentering humanity? Or are there ways to connect these thoughts and approaches to wonder, silence and human flourishing to the question of the global climate change? How does this apophatic and wonder-based thinking interact with the quest to radically transform human lifestyles in order to save the life of "other-than-human'-existences on this planet?

Apophatic wonder, that is, deep contemplative wonder, that create spaces for existential homecoming in ways of being that are of a non-discursive nature, is, we think, connected to deep experiences of entanglement and belonging to nature. There is, we think, an intriguing connection between Environmental Humanities and Health and Medical Humanities.

Health and Medical Humanities helps the doctor or care professional—through liberal arts such as reading poems, listening to music, seeing performative arts, doing philosophical conversations, etc.—to become more human and sensitive towards that which cannot be grasped by medical science and quantitative research methods. Similar connections between Liberal Arts and environmental research are now also being found in the research in environmental humanities. The sense of wonder is indeed seen as key to motivate human beings to act for a more health earth and sustainable societies (Willmott, 2018; Washington, 2019). The sense of wonder helps us to become aware of the inner side of sustainability, or what we will term 'existential sustainability.' This is a dimension which in our view has been overlooked in the research and policy making around United Nations' Seventeen Sustainable Development Goals. In fact, we will today point to a need for an Eighteenth Sustainable Development Goal, which has to do with this existential dimension of sustainability. We see culture, art, philosophy, and spiritual practices as important sources for a radical transformation of human lifestyles in a more sustainable way both in the physical, psychological, sociological, and spiritual way. With a re-humanization of healthcare, education and welfare should also follow a less anthropocentric worldview and a greater awareness of the value of the "other-than-human" life we are a part of.

REFERENCES

Franke, W. (2020). *On the Universality of What Is Not: The Apophatic Turn in Critical Thinking*. Notre Dame, Indiana: University of Notre Dame.

Gadamer, H.-G. (2006). *Truth and Method*. New York: Continuum.

Kohlen, H. (2009). *Conflicts of care: Hospital ethics committees in the USA and Germany*. Campus Verlag.

Marcel, G. (1950). *The Mystery of Being. (Vol. 1: Reflection and Mystery).* Sound Bend, IN: Sct. Augustine's Press.

Rosa, H. (2016). *Resonanz. Eine Soziologie der Weltbeziehung*. Berlin: Suhrkamp.

Rosa, H. (2019: *Unverfügbarkeit*, Vienna: Residenz.

Washington, H. (2019). *A Sense of Wonder Towards Nature. Healing the planet through Belonging*. London: Routledge.

Willmott, G. (2018). *Reading for Wonder: Ecology, Ethics, Enchantment*. New York: Palgrave Macmillan.

Index

About the Contributors

Finn Thorbjørn Hansen is a full professor in applied philosophy at the research section on Arts, Aesthetics, and Health, University of Aalborg, Denmark and PhD in Philosophy of Education, and from 2018–2020 he also owned a Professor II position at the University of Agder. He is the founder of the Danish Society of Philosophical Practice. His main area of research is the phenomenology and ethics of wonder and existential and ethical phenomenology. He has been heading several sponsored action research projects in the area of health, higher education, design, and innovation where so-called 'Wonder Labs' and wonder-based dialogues have been tried out. He has developed a unique form of philosophical and phenomenological action research method. He has written several books on philosophical practice and how these practices can be of relevance to design schools, universities, hospice, hospitals, and public organizations. He also trains professionals in philosophical counseling and Socratic Dialogue Groups and Wonder Labs. https://vbn.aau.dk/en/persons/123561/publications/

Carlo Leget is a full professor of care ethics at the University of Humanistic Studies in Utrecht, the Netherlands. At the same university he holds an endowed chair in palliative care, established by the Netherlands Comprehensive Cancer Organisation (IKNL) and the Association Hospice Care Netherlands (AHZN). His research focuses on the intersection of care, meaning, and end-of-life issues. He is a member of the Health Council of the Netherlands, was vice president of the EAPC from 2012–2019, is a co-founder of the EAPC reference group spirituality, and developed a contemporary model for spiritual care based on the medieval ars moriendi tradition, which is much used and researched in the Netherlands and Belgium. His current research centers around the development of care ethics combined with empirical research with regard to the vulnerability of people in different stages of life, fundamental questions about moral epistemology, and the place of human beings among other life forms in times of ecological crisis.

Solveig Botnen Eide is a full professor of ethics in social work at the University of Oslo, Norway. Her main interest, in both teaching and research, is ethical challenges in professional work. The main themes in her research are ethics and values in child welfare work, ethical challenges in professional conversations and research ethics in practice-oriented research. Her work is inspired by phenomenologically oriented ethics. Her doctoral dissertation deals with ethical challenges in conversations between social workers and children in the child welfare service, with special emphasis on conversations about the children's relationships with their biological mothers.

Åshild Slettebø is a full professor in health science and registered nurse (RN) at Faculty for Health and Sport Sciences, University of Agder, Norway. She holds a PhD in nursing science and ethics. Her main research interests are clinical research within nursing ethics including dignity research, rehabilitation, and research on ethics in the community health care services, in addition to research ethic with experience from Regional and National Committees of Research Ethics in Healthcare and Medicine. In addition, she has research focus on educational research in nursing with a focus on simulation and different approaches to teaching and learning. Her main methodological competence is within different qualitative methods. She is head of the research group 'Healthcare services: Ethics and quality' at the faculty and head of the PhD program at Faculty of Health and Sport Sciences at University of Agder.

Merel Visse (PhD) works in the interdisciplinary fields of care ethics, care theory, and aesthetic inquiry. Her research, writings, and teachings revolve around connecting the arts with central insights of care. She currently leads the Medical and Health Humanities Program at Drew University in Madison, New Jersey, USA. She is also an associate professor at the Care Ethics Department of the University of Humanistic Studies in The Netherlands. www.merelvisse.com

Sine Maria Herholdt-Lomholdt is a registered nurse (RN), Master in Educational Studies, and a PhD in moments of beauty in nursing. She works as an associate professor at faculty of Nursing and Health Sciences at Nord University in Norway. She is the leader of the research group: Caring in Healthcare and affiliated member of the research group: theory of practical knowledge. Her research area are on phenomenology as practice and as research approach as well as philosophic-aesthetical explorations of care practices in nursing.

Aslaug Kristiansen is a full professor of education at the University of Agder, Norway. Her main area of teaching and research are educational theory, ethics, value communication and learning, and dialogue. Her dissertation was a theoretical approach to the issue of trust and trusting relationships within an educational context based on the philosophy of Martin Buber, Knud Løgstrup, Anthony Giddens, and Niklas Luhmann, University of Oslo, 2004.

Claudia Welz founded the Center for the Study of Jewish Thought in Modern Culture at the University of Copenhagen while she was a professor with special responsibilities in Ethics and Philosophy of Religion (2010–2018). Currently, she is a senior research fellow at Forschungskolleg Humanwissenschaften der Goethe-Universität Frankfurt and visiting Professor at University of Duisburg-Essen. She is the author of *Love's Transcendence and the Problem of Theodicy* (2008), *Vertrauen und Versuchung* (2010), *Humanity in God's Image: An Interdisciplinary Exploration* (OUP 2016), and the essay collection *SinnSang: Theologie und Poesie* (2019) about the work of the poet Elazar Benyoëtz. https://claudiawelz.com/cv/

Randi Edland Kroken is a full professor of social work at the University of Agder, Norway. Her main area of teaching and research are child welfare and social work. She focuses on how concrete responsibility in the welfare state is transformed within the system itself. From being a concrete phenomenon at the grassroots level, responsibility appears to turn into something more abstract and liquid at the macro level. She is searching for alternative concepts and language to convey unsayable phenomenon. She edited the book *Omsorgsforståelser. Mellom poesi, profesjon og politikk. (How to understand caring? Between poetry, profession and politics)* (2018). Her main methodological approach is within qualitative methods, and in her writing she seeks to show how social sciences can be combined with human sciences in the field of social work and child welfare.

www.ingramcontent.com/pod-product-compliance
Ingram Content Group UK Ltd.
Pitfield, Milton Keynes, MK11 3LW, UK
UKHW041452071026
15587UKWH00010B/825

9 781666 911206